Skin Wise

A Guide to
Healthy Skin
for Women

Edited by
Annette Callan

Melbourne
OXFORD UNIVERSITY PRESS
Oxford   Auckland   New York

OXFORD UNIVERSITY PRESS AUSTRALIA

Oxford   New York
Athens   Auckland   Bangkok   Bombay
Calcutta   Cape Town   Dar es Salaam   Delhi
Florence   Hong Kong   Istanbul   Karachi
Kuala Lumpur   Madras   Madrid   Melbourne
Mexico City   Nairobi   Paris   Singapore
Taipei   Tokyo   Toronto

and associated companies in
Berlin   Ibadan

OXFORD is a trade mark of Oxford University Press

© Annette Callan, Tanja Bohl, Barbara Breadon, Jill
Cargnello, Gayle Fischer, Anne Howard, Rosemary
Nixon, 1995
First published 1995

This book is copyright. Apart from any fair dealing
for the purposes of private study, research, criticism
or review as permitted under the Copyright Act,
no part may be reproduced, stored in a retrieval
system, or transmitted, in any form or by any means,
electronic, mechanical, photocopying, recording or
otherwise without prior written permission. Enquiries
to be made to Oxford University Press.

Copying for educational purposes
Where copies of part or the whole of the book are
made under Part VB of the Copyright Act, the law
requires that prescribed procedures be followed. For
information, contact the Copyright Agency Limited.

National Library of Australia
Cataloguing-in-Publication data:

Skin wise: a guide to healthy skin for women.

Includes index.
ISBN 0 19 553745 9.

1. Skin — Care and hygiene. 2. Dermatology —
Popular works. I. Callan, Annette.

646.72

Edited by Elaine Cochrane
Indexed by David Suter
Cover design by Cathie Lindsey
Text designed by Steve Randles
Cartoons by Richard G. Dall
Technical illustrations by Juli Kent
Typeset by Desktop Concepts P/L, Melbourne
Printed by SRM Production Services Sdn. Bhd.,
Malaysia
Published by Oxford University Press,
253 Normanby Road, South Melbourne, Australia

CONTENTS

INTRODUCTION
Become skin wise... get to know your skin   v

CHAPTER ONE
Child's play: caring for your child's skin—
it's easy when you know how — Gayle Fischer   1

CHAPTER TWO
A spot of bother: skin problems in adolescence
— Annette Callan   37

CHAPTER THREE
Hormones are a girl's best friend: how hormones
affect our skin from adolescence to old age
— Annette Callan   57

CHAPTER FOUR
Crowning glory: a guide to hair problems
— Jill Cargnello   79

CHAPTER FIVE
Down under: genital skin problems in women
— Tanya Bohl   100

CHAPTER SIX

Your claws are showing: nail problems
— Anne Howard   124

CHAPTER SEVEN

Working girls: skin problems in the workplace
— Rosemary Nixon   132

CHAPTER EIGHT

Why the sun is not a girl's best friend: the sun
and your skin — Rosemary Nixon   142

CHAPTER NINE

Improving on nature: what you can do
to improve your skin
— Barbara Breadon   158

CHAPTER TEN

Light years ahead: lasers for skin problems
— Anne Howard   177

INDEX   183

INTRODUCTION

Become skin wise . . . get to know your skin

Skin Wise is a no-nonsense approach to the understanding of normal skin and some common skin problems that particularly impact on women in their role both as 'skin owners' and as carers of others. It will help you to become skin wise and to know how to care for your skin. It will also help dispel many of the myths surrounding skin care and skin treatment.

Readers will learn about children's skin, including ways to protect young skin from the harmful effects of sunlight and how to help a child if he or she has a skin defect or disease. Also covered are the various problems to which the skin is prone during the hormonally active years from the teens to the menopause. Women's working and home life, as well as their role as child bearers and carers of children, can create further skin problems, and these are discussed in Skin Wise. Also addressed is the changing picture in later life, with the likelihood of skin cancers emerging after a lifetime of sun exposure as well as the general wear-and-tear and the cosmetic deterioration which inevitably accompany ageing.

Probably most women are to some extent dissatisfied with the appearance of their skin. In the pages of glossy magazines, we see young, apparently blemish-free, impossibly slim women. There is not an extra facial or body hair in sight, let alone the odd pimple, blackhead, or burst capillary on the cheeks. This is not reality. The truth is that *normal* skin has imperfections and flaws. Photographs of older women in magazines are usually carefully airbrushed: visible pores, blackheads, fine capillaries, wrinkles and a fine moustache on the upper lip will not sell cosmetics and face creams.

Our skin is our largest, most conspicuous, most vulnerable and at the same time most resilient organ. Its colour and quality are determined by genetic inheritance, so human skins are as infinitely variable as individuals themselves. Like all body organs, the skin alters and deteriorates with age. Far more than internal organs, our skin suffers from the impact of environmental influences. Ultraviolet irradiation, chemicals and toxins in the outside environment, applied cosmetics and medications as well as physical injury all affect the skin. How we care for our skin and the degree of protection we give it may well determine how well it serves us to the end of our life.

Most of us will suffer from a skin problem at some stage in our lives. Because skin is our outer coating, when it malfunctions or develops an abnormality of some kind, it is likely to alter our body image and affect the way in which we interact with others. A disfiguring skin condition does little for our self-esteem.

Skin is not an inert covering for our body. It is an active, constantly changing organ with important roles in the body's day-to-day functions. It provides a protective coating, shielding underlying tissues from the outside environment. It provides a barrier against the penetration of chemicals and microbes, and at the same time blocks loss of water and other vital tissue chemicals from the body to the exterior. It helps our bodies maintain a constant core temperature. We lose

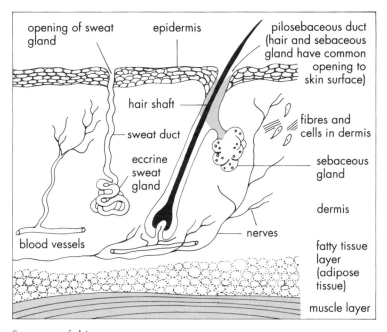

Structure of skin

heat through evaporation of sweat from the surface, and radiate heat when the intricate network of skin blood vessels dilates, thus increasing blood flow through the skin. Heat is conserved when the blood vessels constrict to decrease blood flow through the skin. Myriads of tiny nerve endings and fibres send sensory signals to the brain to give information about the external environment. We register emotions via our skin, flushing in embarrassment and anger, sweating and blanching in fear and shock.

The psyche and skin are closely inter-related. It is not surprising that emotional problems can manifest as skin eruptions. Some of us bite our nails when anxious. An extension of this is fiddling with the hair or hair pulling and even deliberate destructive scratching of the skin. It is small wonder that many skin diseases are worsened by psychological stress. Eczema for example can be precipitated into active phases during stressful periods. Conversely an ugly skin eruption can so affect a person's self-esteem as to create major psychological problems.

Around 2000 skin diseases have been documented. Some of these are so common they have become part of everyday language. Others are so rare that most dermatologists never see them in a lifetime of clinical practice. Skin diseases range from the various benign and malignant skin tumours through infections with various microbes including viruses, bacteria and fungi, to vast numbers of different types of skin inflammations and other eruptions which defy classification.

Our skin, hair and nails play a role in sexual attraction and also say a lot about our general health. Doctors often look for clues in the skin, hair and nails when trying to elucidate various medical problems. Certain skin diseases may be pointers to internal illness—dermatologists are sometimes the first to detect the early manifestation of AIDS, diabetes, thyroid disease or anaemia.

The skin is constructed in two layers of different types of tissue.

The **epidermis** is the outer layer and consists of a compact three-dimensional mosaic of cells. It varies in thickness in different body areas. On the soles of the feet it may be up to 1 mm thick; on areas like the eyelids it is around 0.1 mm thick. The cells of the epidermis are constantly being replaced from the lower layers, gradually moving upwards, changing into flat scales by the time they reach the upper layers and are finally shed from the surface. This transit time varies but is estimated in normal skin as taking one to two months.

The outermost layer of the epidermis, the **stratum corneum**, is particularly thick in areas like the soles of the feet. It consists of flat overlapping scales of a protein substance called **keratin**. Keratin is also the material which constitutes our hair and nails although in these its structure and arrangement are different from that of the stratum corneum.

The lowest layer of the epidermis is called the **basal layer** and consists of cells which have the potential to form new epidermal cells to replace those lost from the surface. Among the cells of the basal layer are also found the pigment forming cells or **melanocytes**. These cells are responsible for forming skin pigment and determine variations in pigmentation between individuals and in different races. All humans of all races and skin colours have the same number of melanocytes, variously estimated as between 1000 and 3000 per square millimetre depending on the area of skin. The difference between dark skin and pale skin is in the amount of pigment produced and in the arrangement and distribution of the pigment throughout the epidermis.

The lower layer of skin is the **dermis**. This is a much thicker layer and comprises the supporting framework of our skin, giving its elasticity, resilience and strength. These properties are mainly due to a framework of cunningly arranged fibres known as **collagen** and **elastin**, embedded in a jelly-like substance. It also contains numerous types of individual cells, all of which have important functions. The dermis also contains networks of fine skin **nerves**. Some delicate nerve fibres pierce the lower layers of the epidermis and they also surround hair follicles, allowing us to feel sensations like touch, heat, cold, pain and itch. The nourishment of the skin is taken care of by its rich network of tiny blood vessels bringing oxygen, nutrients, and the hormones which affect growth and metabolism of our skin. *The skin cannot be nourished or fed from the outside.*

Underneath the dermis is the **subcutaneous tissue** containing the fat (**adipose tissue**). This functions as a protective and cushioning layer and varies in thickness in various body areas. It is absent altogether in some sites such as the eyelid. Adipose tissue has an active metabolism and is a very important tissue for hormone activity.

Our skin is pierced by two kinds of pores. The minuscule sweat pores are not visible to the naked eye but sweat emerges through them from underlying coiled, tubular **sweat glands** situated in the dermis. Sweat glands are found over the entire body surface but are most numerous on the palms and soles. The other skin pore is the combined opening of the oil or **sebaceous gland** and the **hair follicle.** The oily substance (**sebum**) produced by sebaceous glands works its way from the gland into the upper part of the long tubular canal containing the hair, and hence reaches the surface through the same opening. These pores are called **pilo-sebaceous follicles.** Although hairs are visible over much of the body surface, the sebaceous glands are usually inconspicuous except on areas like the nose where they are rather prominent in adult skin.

The skin surface is coated with a film consisting of a mixture of sebum, sweat and other substances which result from the chemical breakdown of surface cells. This film is slightly acidic and is called the **acid mantle.** If anything disrupts this slight acidity, healthy skin is capable of adjusting it back to normal levels very quickly. Maintenance of this slight acidity used to be thought important for protection against the penetration of harmful microbes. The constant sloughing of dead cells from the skin surface, known as exfoliation, which is constantly occurring at an invisible level, is now regarded as the most important means of not allowing microbes to gain a foothold on the surface of healthy skin.

The above simplified description of the structure and function of our skin does scant justice to a marvellous and intricate human organ, but it will help you to understand what follows in this book. Remember that 'normal skin' as defined by advertising agencies and the media is not reality. Skin which performs all its physiological functions adequately and whose appearance is consistent with a person's age and ethnic background is normal from the medical point of view. If, in addition, it has an aesthetically pleasant appearance, then this is a bonus. The skin is at its best in childhood when it is unlined and lacks obvious pores and is covered in most areas in fine hairs. This must alter as we grow into adulthood and, unfortunately, the definition of normal skin as decreed by the media falls well short of reality. No skin is completely free of small blemishes, alterations in texture and colour, minor irritations and prominent pores, and it is time we started to object strongly to the definition of normality imposed on us by the cosmetic and advertising industries. Beauty is indeed more than skin deep!

CHAPTER ONE

CHILD'S PLAY

Caring for your child's skin —

it's easy when you know how

GAYLE FISCHER

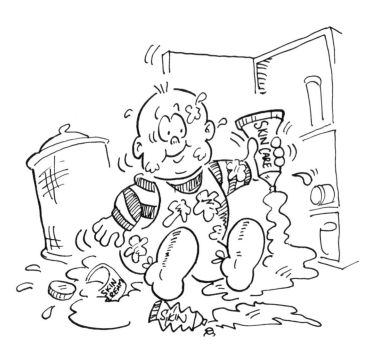

Perfect babies have perfect skin, but *real* babies and children have blotches and bumps, itches and rashes, some minor, some more serious. Sun protection, or lack of it, can affect skin health for the rest of the child's life, and some skin conditions that trouble adults, such as psoriasis, may first appear in childhood.

BIRTHMARKS

A 'birthmark' is any unusual mark on the surface of the skin that turns up early in life and is then there for good. They are very common, normal, and mostly small and harmless.

Despite the name, birthmarks aren't always present at birth and can appear at any time during childhood. Once there they are usually permanent, but their appearance and colour can change with time.

From a skin specialist's point of view birthmarks are very diverse and complex. They are made of many different elements that are normally in the skin, but which in this case are present in excess. They are grouped according to what they are made of, be it blood vessels, pigment cells, or other things such as glands or hair.

Birthmarks are not all the same. There are many different appearances and types, shapes and sizes. In most cases they are best left alone because they don't cause any trouble. Sometimes, however, they can be dangerous in themselves or can be linked to other abnormalities that are dangerous. Also, some parents are anxious to have them removed to improve their child's appearance. This is often much easier said than done. If your child has a birthmark it's worth having it checked out to make sure that it is one of the harmless kinds.

Discussing all the different types of birthmarks would take up this whole book and wouldn't be worth it as many are very rare. Let's consider some of the more common ones.

Birthmarks consisting of blood vessels

Many birthmarks consist of networks or clusters of tiny blood vessels visible just under the surface of the skin.

Stork marks (naevus flammeus)

'Stork marks' are the commonest of all birthmarks, occurring in 50 per cent of newborn babies. They look like red blotches on the forehead, bridge of the nose, eyelids and nape of the neck. When the baby cries they look redder than ever. They are usually trivial, but sometimes are quite extensive. They certainly aren't anything to worry about. They don't bother your baby and the ones on the face always disappear by the time the child is one, often before. The ones on the nape of the neck are often permanent, but this doesn't matter as they will be covered by hair.

Strawberry marks (haemangioma)

This is another very common birthmark, seen in 10–20 per cent of all babies. They are a little more common in premature babies. Usually there is only one, but sometimes several are present. Although they can already be there on the day the baby is born, it is more usual for the perfect new baby to develop them suddenly in the first few weeks of life. They start as a red or sometimes white patch that rapidly grows into a rounded bump which is usually bright red, hence the name 'strawberry'. This old fashioned name isn't quite accurate, however, as some haemangiomas are blue or purple. No matter what colour they are, they all behave the same way.

Haemangiomas are seen most often on the face, scalp and trunk, but they can occur anywhere. After they appear, they grow for a few weeks to months, usually to no more than a centimetre or two across. They then remain the same for a very variable length of time, sometimes months, sometimes years. Eventually they all disappear, usually without a trace or with just a faint red mark. This happens by the time the child is in primary school.

Most haemangiomas don't cause any trouble at all, and because we can expect them to vanish by themselves, the best thing to do is to leave them alone. However they can occasionally be a problem if they are very large, if they are on the face, or if they are near the eye where they can stop the baby from seeing properly. If they are under the nappy, friction can cause them to ulcerate and this can be a problem too. Doctors usually assess troublesome haemangiomas with an ultrasound examination, which is safe and painless. Haemangiomas causing problems can be treated. Because treatment usually involves using cortisone, and sometimes laser therapy, we need to have a very good reason for treating them.

If your child is one of many with a haemangioma there is usually nothing at all to worry about, and it's best to let nature take its course.

Port wine stains (capillary malformation)

Port wine stains are a much less common birthmark, occurring in only about one in a thousand babies. The mark is always there at birth, and this is because it is formed very early in life, probably in the first trimester of pregnancy. It's not a growth which will disappear like a haemangioma, but a permanent part of the baby that will always stay the same, unless it is removed.

A port wine stain is a completely flat pink-to-red blotch with a well defined edge at birth. They are nearly always just on one side of the body. They can occur anywhere on the skin. At birth they are often so faint that they aren't even noticed, but they become brighter with time, and in adults can look purple and become lumpy.

Port wine stains occur because of excessive formation of blood vessels in parts of the baby's skin during pregnancy. We don't know why this happens and it certainly isn't anything that the mother did wrong, it's just bad luck. Nevertheless, because there is an error present, the mark on the skin can just be the tip of the iceberg, and there may be other things wrong underneath. This is particularly the case if the port wine stain is on the face and involves the upper eyelid, in which case there may be something wrong with the eye and sometimes the brain. These birthmarks, particularly if extensive, should always be checked by a doctor.

Because port wine stains will not disappear by themselves, treatment is desirable if they are on a visible part of the skin. The best treatment for these birthmarks at present is laser therapy, which is now available in most capital cities in Australia. As it is painful it is done with the aid of a general anaesthetic. It can be carried out early in the child's life, and ideally should be completed before he or she starts pre-school.

Birthmarks consisting of pigment cells

Brown birthmarks (congenital melanocytic naevi)

This is another fairly common birthmark, present at birth in one in a hundred babies. Sometimes they can also appear in the first one to two years of life. These birthmarks, unlike the ones described already, are made of melanocytes, the cells in the skin that normally make brown pigment.

Brown birthmarks are usually single and small, less than a centimetre in diameter at birth. Unless they are on the face, they don't cause much concern, and most people can accept them as quite usual. Sometimes, however, they can be very large, to the extent of covering most of the nappy area, in which case they are called 'bathing trunk naevi'. Fortunately, this is very rare, but it's not unusual to have one that is several centimetres in length. With time they may become hairy, and later in childhood and early adolescence, lumpy as well.

There are two concerns with brown birthmarks. The first is that they are unattractive, and the second is that there is a risk that they may become malignant. We don't know how great the risk of malignancy really is, because so far we don't have any really long-term studies to give us this information, but it's estimated to be about one to two per cent over a whole lifetime. It is certainly very rare for malignancy to occur in a brown birthmark before puberty, but the larger the birthmark the greater the chance is thought to be.

For both these reasons, parents often choose to have brown birthmarks removed. Sometimes this can be done easily, if they are small. However, if they are large, removing them can be a very difficult and drawn-out process involving many operations. The end result is sometimes as unattractive as the original birthmark! It's therefore not an easy decision to go ahead with such an undertaking and needs very careful consideration, with lots of discussion taking place between parents, skin specialist and surgeon. A small brown birthmark is probably best left in place until just before puberty as the risk of malignancy is negligible, and at the age of 11 or 12 the child can have some role in the decision about whether to remove it or not. Of course if a child is terribly embarrassed by the look of one of these birthmarks, particularly if it is on the face, then it's very reasonable to consider having it removed earlier.

Mongolian spots

These birthmarks are rarely seen in Caucasian babies (that is babies with European ancestry), but are very common in Asian babies. They occur on the back and shoulders and are present at birth. They look like brown or black oval stains on the skin. They are quite harmless and don't have any tendency to become malignant. Very often they disappear early in childhood. Because they occur on parts of the skin that aren't usually seen, and because they usually go away, no treatment is needed.

ECZEMA

Eczema, or dermatitis (these are two words that mean exactly the same thing), is the commonest skin problem seen in childhood. The tendency to suffer from eczema, asthma or hay fever is inherited, that is, passed from one generation to the next. People with the tendency are described as *atopic*. It is estimated that 10–20 per cent of the Australian population is atopic, but it takes more than just the inherited tendency to produce an illness—you need the right (or wrong!) environment as well. This is because atopic people are allergic to many things in the environment which set off their condition and if they aren't exposed to them they won't have a problem.

The first sign of eczema usually occurs in the first six months of life, although it can start at any time in childhood or even as an adult. Parents notice that their baby has a rough, dry skin, often with red scaly patches on the face and the creases of the elbows and knees. These children feel very itchy, and although they may be too young to scratch, they let you know they are uncomfortable by becoming unsettled and sleeping poorly. This can be very disturbing for everyone in the house. Later on they do start scratching and do this as soon as their clothes are removed and they are able to reach their skin. This produces raw areas on the skin surface that are then prone to infection.

Many people believe that eczema is something that you grow out of. This certainly can happen, but a child who has had eczema may always have a dry, irritable skin that needs extra care, and if environmental conditions are not right the eczema may resurface. So although you can live in hope, it's not a good idea to assume that the problem will go away completely.

So what can you do if your child has eczema? The first thing to remember is that you are not alone—it's a very common problem that lots of people successfully learn to take in their stride, but it does mean daily chores for you and your child. Eczema is something that can't be cured, but this *doesn't* mean that nothing can be done. It *does* mean that the eczema has to be controlled on a day-to-day basis, and this means never giving up or getting lazy. Parents often feel frustrated because when they treat their child the problem goes away, only to show up again when they stop treatment. They take this to mean that treatment has been a failure, and this simply isn't true. What it does mean is that treatment is aimed at keeping the problem at bay and that it was working. We can't make the problem go away, because we can't change the inherited makeup of the child. It's very important to accept this as soon as possible, because once you do it will help you to help your child. It's hard at first, but once you are in a daily routine of skin care, its amazing how easy it can become.

What does all this actually involve? The first thing is to deal with things in the environment that might irritate your child's skin. One of the commonest of these is soap—this irritates sensitive skin. Your chemist should be able to recommend non-soap alternatives, or you can improvise by washing with moisturising cream, or just swirl an old stocking filled with oatmeal in the bath. Avoid bubble bath and anything that foams. The best thing to add to the bath is dispersable bath oil (not 'baby oil').

It's also important to look at what your child is wearing. Ideally children with eczema should be dressed in pure cotton or cotton blends with about 70 per cent cotton. Synthetics and wool will aggravate their skin. Of course clothes are only one way that they come into contact with these fabrics. Look out for woollen car-seat covers, blankets, toys, carpets and sheepskins, not to mention wool that you are wearing yourself as you carry your child. You may need to be creative in thinking of ways to substitute or cover woollen objects so that they don't make contact with the child's skin.

Ask yourself also what your child is making contact with in the backyard, at pre-school or school, or at the beach or pool. Direct skin contact with sand should be avoided. Some children have problems sitting on a very dusty floor, or rolling in the grass. Some are irritated by contact with pets. Hobby materials such as craft glue and paints may harm sensitive hands. Chlorinated water can dry out the skin and may need to be rinsed off as soon as the child comes out of the pool.

There are some things in the environment which will make eczema worse that are just beyond your control! Cold, dry windy conditions don't suit some children, while others are worse when its hot and humid. Similarly dust and mould levels are often hard to control despite the most meticulous cleaning routines. You just have to live with this, and step up your treatment routine accordingly.

What about allergy? Parents always ask this question, and its a very relevant one, considering that children with eczema, when tested, are often allergic to various foods and airborne substances. If you suspect a food allergy it's worth having this checked out, but please don't restrict your child's diet without making sure from an expert that his or her nutrition will still be adequate. Allergy testing may tell you what your child is allergic to—some of it can be avoided, some is in the impossible-to-avoid group. However, avoidance of allergens is rarely the whole answer with eczema, and is not a substitute for careful, daily skin care.

Skin care

Care of an eczema sufferer's skin involves the use of creams and ointments. It's time consuming and children aren't always terribly cooperative about it, particularly when it involves treating their faces. It's important to make it as much fun as possible, and to involve children from the beginning in their own treatment. Often they like smearing cream around and this is fine as long as you make sure it goes on the right places! Combining treatment with another activity such as a favourite TV show or story can also be helpful.

Children with eczema have dry, rough skins. They don't retain moisture well and you need to make up for this by applying moisturising creams. These should go all over the skin a couple of times a day, sometimes more. In addition to this, most skin specialists would also recommend a cortisone cream to use on areas of active eczema. Sometimes creams and ointments can cause stinging, especially if the skin is very raw. If this happens, it's important to let your doctor know so a substitute can be recommended.

A word about cortisone creams. Many parents are frightened to use cortisone creams on their children. They have heard from their friends, neighbours, relatives, chemist and just about anybody they care to ask that they are very dangerous. This is simply not true. If used *correctly* on the right areas of the body and in the amounts that your doctor recommends they are in fact very safe. It's true that they can damage the skin, but *only* if they are used to excess. This is highly unlikely to happen as most parents are so cautious about using them. One of the commonest mistakes parents make in treating their children is to under-utilise their cortisone creams, or to put off using them until their child is in a real mess. The end result is poorly controlled eczema, an itchy irritable child, and eventually more rather than less cortisone being required. It's important to get things in perspective and to recognise the benefits of cortisone as opposed to the risks, and in the case of eczema the benefits outweigh the risks by a long way!

There are other things which your child with eczema may need from time to time. Antibiotics may be needed if the skin becomes infected. Antihistamines that can be bought over the counter aren't much use, and often make children drowsy or, even worse, overexcited. Evening primrose oil is a 'natural therapy' which has been recommended for eczema, and sometimes it seems to work, but it isn't always successful. Before embarking on any therapy that involves your child taking medicine by mouth it's wise to check with your doctor.

If your child has been diagnosed as having eczema it certainly is not a disaster. Even the minority of children with severe eczema can be well controlled, provided you and your child get into a regular daily routine of avoiding the things that irritate the skin and using your creams correctly.

CRADLE CAP

Cradle cap is a persistently scaly scalp, seen quite often in babies and pre-school children. The scaling usually affects the crown, but sometimes can be seen over the entire scalp. The scale is thick and white, and not easily picked off.

Cradle cap is not a diagnosis, as there are three common skin conditions that can affect the scalp in this way. The most frequent cause in small babies is a condition called **seborrhoeic dermatitis**. This is a red, scaly rash that affects the scalp, face, nappy area and skin folds. Although it looks dramatic, it does not cause the baby any discomfort and usually fades away by the time the baby is about six months old. Cradle cap may also be the first sign of psoriasis, or occasionally it may be part of atopic dermatitis (eczema), but in these children there is usually obvious dermatitis elsewhere on the skin.

Seborrhoeic dermatitis is not seen in children over a year old. Psoriasis is the commonest cause of cradle cap in these older children, particularly if they don't have eczema elsewhere on their skin, although other signs of psoriasis may never appear.

Whatever the cause of cradle cap, treatment is much the same. If it is mild, the excess scale can be removed by massaging baby oil into the scalp and then shampooing. A plain moisturising cream can then be applied. If this is not effective, prescription medication is available from your doctor. A severe case should certainly be seen by a doctor, because the cause may be psoriasis.

Just as a mild degree of dandruff is common in adults (see page 83), it is not uncommon for children to have a scaly scalp from time to time. Many cases of cradle cap are very mild, do not represent any particular skin disease, and do not require any treatment at all.

WARTS

Did you know that warts are caused by a virus? Viruses cause infections—things like the common cold, chicken pox and measles. Viruses cause many different symptoms. The one that gives you warts makes lumps appear on your skin. Warts can appear anywhere on the skin and also on the lips, genital area and even inside the mouth. They can be any size from a pinhead to several centimetres across.

In children, the commonest places for warts are on the hands, knees and feet. Warts around the nails can be a real problem and warts on the soles of the feet, **plantar warts**, can be painful. It's also not uncommon for children to get spiky warts on their nostrils or lips. These are called **filiform** warts. Less commonly they may get dozens of tiny warts, called **plane** warts, on their hands and faces.

Warts can occur around the anus and genital area in children, usually because the child has warts on the hands and they have been transferred there by scratching. Warts can also be sexually acquired, and this means that a child who has been sexually abused can get warts this way. Sexual abuse is a very serious problem and if you suspect that it may have happened to your child you should seek help from your doctor or community health service immediately.

In general, warts are quite harmless. As with the majority of viruses, the body's own defence mechanisms eventually rid us of the problem. In most children this happens within a couple of years, sometimes more quickly, sometimes more slowly, but it does usually happen. After they are gone, they rarely become a big problem again.

The best thing to do with warts in children, especially if they aren't causing a problem, is to ignore them, and they'll eventually go away without a trace. If they are causing pain and embarrassment, and particularly if your child is keen for you to do something about them, there are numerous things that you can try. In fact just about everyone has their own favourite remedy for warts! You'll hear about banana skins and chickweed, hypnotherapy and people 'buying warts' for 20 cents. In many cases it may just be that the treatment was used just as the warts were about to go away anyway. Some people believe it's mind over matter. A more scientific explanation is that, if you can damage a wart in some way, this will enable the body's immune system to recognise that it's not meant to be there and destroy it, and hopefully all the other warts with it.

Wart paints and plasters are available from the chemist, many without a prescription. Be careful when using them, and follow instructions carefully, as sometimes they can be irritating to the skin.

If all this fails, you can see your doctor about having warts removed. This is best done by freezing them as surgical methods involving burning or cutting may leave scarring. Remember also that children tolerate painful procedures poorly. They may remember the experience for a long time, even into adulthood, and it can make them scared of the doctor afterwards. It is also sadly true that just about every method ever described for eradicating warts has a considerable failure rate, and this means that your child may go through a painful procedure only to have the warts come back again. So its important to give it a lot of thought before you go ahead, and keep in mind that if you let the warts resolve of their own accord that they will do so painlessly, and without leaving any marks.

PSORIASIS

Psoriasis is a skin condition which affects one in every hundred people. It is inherited, and this means that parents pass it on to their children, just as they might pass on blue eyes or red hair. It's not an infection, and no one can catch it from you, but if your child has inherited it from you, he or she may pass it on to their children as well.

Skin is continually renewing itself. It has to be able to do this because, being on the outside, it's so easily injured. Psoriasis comes about because of a tendency for this renewal process to occur too quickly. As a result the skin doesn't have a chance to achieve its normal mature, smooth surface and instead looks red and scaly. Sometimes its also itchy and even sore. The abnormal areas fortunately rarely involve the whole skin. It's more common for them to occur in patches here and there.

In adults psoriasis can be associated with arthritis, and this is said to occur in up to 10 per cent of patients. Mild skin disease can be associated with severe arthritis, and sometimes it isn't realised for years that a patient has psoriatic arthritis until they develop the typical rash.

Psoriasis can occur on any part of the skin, including the scalp and around the genital area. It can also affect the nails. It is unusual for it to start in childhood. The average time is in the 20s. However it certainly can be seen much earlier, even in babies.

When psoriasis appears for the first time in childhood it is often quite different to the way adults experience it. In babies it may appear to be just a difficult nappy rash or cradle cap. Older children often have rashes on their scalp or behind their ears. Sometimes a sore throat or a bout of tonsillitis can be followed by an attack of small red scaly spots that then lasts a few weeks. A child who also has a tendency to eczema, which is much more common in childhood than psoriasis, may have a rash that has characteristics of both.

Fortunately, if psoriasis does start in childhood it is usually quite mild, but children can sometimes be severely affected. It is however rare for them to experience arthritis.

It is important to realise that the reason a person has psoriasis is purely because it is imprinted on their genetic makeup. It is not an allergy or an infection or a vitamin deficiency. And unfortunately it can't be cured once it has started. This doesn't mean a hopeless situation! For the majority with psoriasis, it is a minor nuisance only, and may sometimes disappear for long periods. As with eczema its usually a simple matter to control it with creams and ointments, particularly in children.

Psoriasis is a very unpredictable condition. Sometimes in a person's life it is trivial, and at other times severe. One of the things that tends to make it worse is stress of any kind, either physical or emotional, and this is why, in children, it may surface after an infection, or after emotional trauma.

Unlike eczema, there is no need to go to a lot of trouble to modify your child's environment if he or she has psoriasis. Skin specialists don't believe that diet has any effect on it, nor are special washing products or clothing required. Perhaps the only preventative measure that one could take as a parent would be to minimise emotional stress in your child's life as much as possible. We all try to do this of course, but any parent will tell you that it's much easier said than done.

If you suspect that your child may have psoriasis, especially if there is a history of it in the family, you should see your doctor. This is because the treatment of psoriasis is complex and must be individualised to each patient. Don't assume that because someone else in the family was severely affected that your child will be too. The diagnosis of psoriasis rarely signifies disaster! Like all chronic conditions it takes a while to come to terms with. Every patient experiences this in a different way and the more accepting and positive you are about it, the easier it is on you and your child.

MOLES—ARE THEY DANGEROUS?

People often worry a lot about their moles. Will they become cancerous? Should they all be removed just in case? Why are they there at all?

Moles are completely normal—everyone has them, although we don't all have the same type and number.

Occasionally, a mole will be present at birth (see brown birthmarks). It's much more common, however, for them to appear after the age of two or three. At about this time you will notice small brown, fawn or reddish spots and lumps occurring on your child's skin. Often they seem to come up over night. They can occur anywhere on the skin surface, including the scalp. Once present, they grow slowly with your child.

There are two main concerns that people have about moles. One is that they may turn into a dangerous type of cancer called a melanoma. The other is that they don't look nice. The first concern is obviously much more important from a medical point of view.

Let's take the first concern first. How do you know if a mole has become a cancer? Something that isn't well under-stood about moles is that they have a life of their own, inde-pendent of yours! After appearing in childhood they grow and change slowly over your lifetime, and eventually disap-pear when you're old. New moles tend to appear right through childhood, adolescence and even in early adult-hood, and occasionally even in middle life, although this is unusual. If you only look at your moles about once every year or two, don't be surprised if they have changed. They may have turned a different colour or shape, or grown or shrunk in size. They may have developed a ring of a differ-ent colour around them. Some may have disappeared. All of this is normal.

There are two times in life when these changes are partic-ularly prominent. One is in childhood when growth is rapid, and the other is during pregnancy.

If a mole changes rapidly it often causes alarm. Some changes that happen virtually over night, such as sudden swelling or darkening, usually mean that the mole has been knocked or twisted. This usually recovers rapidly. A change that happens a little more slowly but is still noticeable over a period of weeks or months is the one that you have to worry about. This is particularly true of changes in colour, shape, size and thickness that make the mole look asymmetrical or different from all your other moles. Bleeding, particularly if it happens on more than one occasion, or persistent itching are also cause for concern.

Sometimes, particularly in childhood, a mole can become itchy or irritable, develop a symmetrical white ring around it and then fade or disappear. This can sometimes happen to several moles at once. This is called the halo naevus phenomenon and is completely harmless. It just means that your body has decided for whatever reason to remove the mole, and with it goes some surrounding pigmentation as well.

Is anyone more at risk for getting a melanoma than others? We do know that in some cases, melanoma seems to run in families. We also know that excess sun exposure plays some role, as sunny climates such as Australia have very high rates of melanoma. People with very fair skins, and those with lots of moles are also at greater risk than others.

It's important, and also reassuring, to know that malignant change in moles is particularly rare in childhood, although after puberty it does rise toward adult figures. If you are concerned about your child's moles there are two things you should be doing. One is careful sun protection. (See 'Sun-protecting your child', page 23.) The other is watching the moles yourself. (See page 150.) It's best to do this every two to three months or so, and it can be helpful to have some photographs to jog your memory. If you inspect the moles every day you will not spot changes. If you look very infrequently, you will see lots of changes, and probably all the changes will be normal, but they may alarm you unnecessarily. Don't rely solely on a yearly checkup by the doctor. Take some responsibility yourself, just as you might do with regular breast self-examination.

Even though it's had lots of publicity, and many people seem to have known or heard of some young person who has had a melanoma, it's still a relatively rare event. It's wise to be cautious, but don't worry too much!

What about that second concern, that moles don't look nice? Teenagers are often particularly worried about this. Certainly if a great big black mole turns up right on the tip of your nose you would have every justification in wanting it removed. But most moles are on the trunk and legs, and even though you may not like them, the fact is that they do look natural. Moles are seen in everyone and other people expect you to have them. In fact, although you may be self-conscious about them, other people probably barely notice them. The same cannot be said of scars, and it is very hard to remove a mole, especially from the trunk, without producing a scar. Sometimes scars can be very obvious indeed, and can remain itchy and tender for months after the mole has been removed. Unlike moles, scars don't look natural, and other people are much more likely to notice them and ask you about them than they do with moles.

Unless a mole has changed in a worrying way, looks very unusual, or is so unpleasant-looking that a scar would be an improvement, its best to leave it where it is. Having all your moles removed, just in case, just isn't worth it! This is particularly true in childhood, when the operation involved would nearly always involve a general anaesthetic. This is because most children would find it difficult and disturbing to have it done with a local anaesthetic, which involves a needle, and can be very frightening.

Do remember the low risk of moles in childhood. If you are concerned that a mole should be removed, discuss it with your doctor, and make sure you know all the risks of the operation before you go ahead.

Nappy rash

Nappy rash is a form of dermatitis which affects the area under the nappy. It probably affects most babies in a minor form at some time or another, but some babies tolerate nappies poorly and seem to be plagued by it all the time. It's not really surprising that the skin in this location gets irritated. Imagine what your bottom would be like if you went around all day wearing a hot, wet towel and a pair of plastic pants!

The commonest reason for nappy rash is just irritation from the wet, urine-soaked nappy, but there can be other reasons as well. Sometimes a baby may get an infection in this area, most often with thrush. An illness which causes diarrhoea or high fevers can result in nappy rash, because this increases heat and wetness under the nappy. Sometimes persistent nappy rashes can be the first sign of psoriasis.

Many parents and health care professionals are convinced that teething causes nappy rash. Not all doctors agree, and if it is true, nobody knows why. Fortunately, like most things which stir up the skin under the nappy, this is of finite duration!

Treating nappy rash is pretty straightforward. The first thing to do is to take all the lotions, powders and potions you've been using to treat it and throw them out. Keep it as simple as you can. The more things you put on the tender skin, the worse you may make it, and you may even be using something that your baby is allergic to.

Remember that nappy rash happens because the skin is overheated and wet. So you have to aim at the opposite of this—dry and cool. How do you do this? A simple way is to use good quality disposable nappies which contain material that traps urine below the surface of the nappy. If, however, you have concerns about the cost or the environmental impact of disposable nappies, or you just feel its a huge waste of that huge, snowy white pile of cloth nappies you own, then you can modify the way you are using your cloth nappies to overcome the nappy rash.

Using cloth nappies usually means a whole lot of other paraphernalia. Plastic pants, nappy liners and fluffy overpants all make it easier to clean the nappies and stop them leaking, but if you are going to get your baby over an attack of nappy rash you'll have to give them a miss for a while, as the overpants keep the nappy area too hot and damp, and the nappy liners can be irritating when pressed up against the skin. It's also important to change the nappy as soon as it becomes wet. Some doctors tell mothers simply to leave the nappies off and this is great if it's summer and you are staying at home, preferably away from the carpet, but it can be very impractical advice, so don't feel bad if you just can't manage it.

Some people compromise, and use disposables just for going out or overnight, when it's not so easy to change frequently, and a cloth nappy would get really wet. It's best to be open-minded about nappies if your child has a nappy rash problem. Try different options and different brands of disposables too. Some mothers are convinced that their baby does best in cloth and others swear by disposables. You'll have to experiment.

What about the things you are putting on the skin? Remember that nappy rash is dermatitis (see 'Eczema' (atopic dermatitis), page 6) and the same principles apply. Firstly avoid irritating things on the skin. Cut out soap and use some bath oil (not baby oil) in the bath. At change time, don't use baby wipes. Carry a damp washer with you in a plastic bag, and use a simple non-perfumed moisturiser as a change lotion. After cleaning up, apply a bit more moisturiser to the skin. Avoid things that tend to cake on the skin, such as powders or thick gooey creams, as they just increase dampness and heat. And forget the concept of 'barrier' creams! There really isn't any cream that will protect the skin enough to allow you to forget about keeping it dry by the methods outlined already.

If these strategies just aren't enough, your doctor may prescribe some mild cortisone cream or ointment. This is in keeping with treatment of dermatitis generally. Anti-infective creams may be needed as well, if your doctor feels that infection is playing some role. If you find that your child has a problem with nappy rash that just isn't going away, do see your doctor. Some little ones never seem to have a perfect bottom until they are right out of nappies, and may even have some minor problems even when they are down to night nappies only. And you, as a parent, may have to accept some compromise. As long as your child is comfortable, that's the main thing, and a bit of redness under the nappy is just best ignored.

HOW TO LOOK AFTER ACNE-PRONE SKIN

Acne is a very common skin condition. About half of all teenagers suffer from it. Like many other things that affect the skin, it's a built-in tendency that is part of your genetic make-up, and most young people with acne have a relative who has it as well.

Acne happens because of an abnormality of the **pilo-sebaceous apparatus.** This complex structure in the skin consists of the hair root, to which is attached an oil-producing gland, called the sebaceous gland. In acne this gland makes an oversupply of oil which is unable to easily escape from the skin because the opening of the gland is blocked by a buildup of surface scale. This blockage may become so severe that oil ruptures into the skin, causing redness and swelling. In addition to this there is an overgrowth of bacteria, which seems to play a role as well. It's a very complicated process.

What we see in acne is blackheads, whiteheads, red lumps and yellow pinheads containing pus. Usually it's a mixture of all these different things. The severity ranges from very minor to very disfiguring, but of course teenagers vary enormously in how they perceive this. Some are untroubled, but most of them are pretty embarrassed and would do just about anything to have clear skin.

People usually think that acne is something that just affects teenagers. For the most part they're right, but sometimes it can also affect babies and children. For the acne tendency to express itself, it is necessary to have some androgen, or male hormone, present in the system to stimulate the sebaceous glands which are central to the problem. (This is discussed further in chapter 2.) Male hormone is present in both sexes, although in much larger amounts in men. For the first six months or so of a baby's life, there may be just enough, left over from when he was inside the womb, to cause acne. After this acne is not usually seen again until about the age of eight, when some children begin to mature sexually. At this stage a small amount of male hormone is made which may be just enough to set acne off. If acne is seen between these ages, doctors usually worry that there may be something wrong that is causing excessive amounts of male hormone. However this is very rare.

Acne in babies and pre-pubertal children usually requires only minimal treatment. However at puberty it may sometimes become a lot more severe, and continue to become more of a problem for several years, before resolving in late teenage years or early in the twenties.

As acne is so common it is not surprising that there are lots of old wives' tales about it. The commonest myths are that it is due to lack of cleanliness and that it is due to diet—both totally inaccurate! These and other misconceptions about acne are discussed in chapter 2.

Babies with acne usually don't need any treatment. The acne is usually very mild and goes away by six months or so. If treatment is desired, your doctor can prescribe a mild lotion. Later on in childhood, if the tendency is only to have a few pimples, the acne should be treatable with simple products obtainable from the chemist.

As with most things to do with skin, it's best to keep it simple. Remember you can't wash the problem away. Cleansers, toners, masks and facials will only cost money and do very little in the long run. Simple soap and water is fine to wash the face. Similarly, steaming the face in an attempt to deep-cleanse it will only make the situation worse.

It is important to be aware that greasy products, particularly cosmetics, moisturisers and sunblocks, will aggravate acne and cause pimples. Teenagers often use thick pancake makeup to hide the problem, and unfortunately this causes even more pimples. Try to select oil-free or water-based products. Many of these are available through chemists, department stores and even supermarkets. Sunblocks are available as lotions and gels. These are the best products for acne-prone skin, and don't have to cost a lot of money.

Picking and squeezing should be avoided as much as possible. They usually only prolong the acne lesions, and this may result in permanent scarring. Unfortunately, this can become quite a habit and breaking it takes real willpower. Sometimes the picking may also be a sign of stress, and you may have to look closely at what is really worrying your child.

Don't worry too much about diet. If you are sure that chocolate, or any other food for that matter, always produces a flare up of the acne, by all means cut it out, but no special diet is going to make much difference. A healthy, balanced diet is all your child needs.

Finally, what can you buy from the chemist that can help? The most reliable over-the-counter creams are those that contain an antiseptic called benzoyl peroxide. This goes under various brand names, and comes in several different strengths. Its wise to start with the weakest one and work up. There are also many different acne washes that contain antiseptics, but these aren't necessary if you are using creams. If these are ineffective, particularly if the acne is severe, it's wise to see your doctor, as most other acne treatments are only available on prescription.

When you do see your doctor, he or she will have a range of options to offer you as treatment for acne. Many of these involve swallowing tablets. Acne is, by and large, not a curable condition, but it is nearly always possible to control it with adequate treatment. This may have to be continued for some years, as long as it takes the acne to 'burn out', so some acne treatments can involve being on medicine for a long time. Naturally, this often makes parents nervous, and they worry terribly about the dangers of long-term medication.

Many parents, especially those who themselves didn't have acne and didn't experience the embarrassment of it, feel that it's a natural part of being a teenager and doesn't require treatment. But just ask the teenagers who have the problem how they feel! They'll usually say 'just show me what to do and I'll do it, and I don't care about the dangers'. Parents, on the other hand, often focus only on the dangers. The answer lies somewhere between the two points of view.

If you are a parent of a child with acne, please try to understand how he or she feels. It would be wonderful if it could all be treated with natural measures. But if you have already tried all the strategies outlined above and the acne just isn't responding, you may have to keep an open mind about the value of medication in helping the problem. The acne treatments we have available now are very good and very safe. Remember it does wonders for a teenager's self-esteem to look as good as possible, and you must weigh up the importance of that against your apprehension about medication.

Fortunately, for most sufferes, acne is rarely so severe that it requires a visit to the skin specialist or even the doctor. Although it may last a few years, the tendency is for the worst of it to be over by the end of the teens. But please seek help if your child is distressed by it. It's a very treatable condition! Modern treatment strategies are discussed in chapter 2.

SUN-PROTECTING YOUR CHILD

We live in a very sunny climate, and are all exposed to a lot of sun. Australians have one of the highest skin cancer rates in the world, due almost entirely to our outdoor lifestyle. This isn't to say that we shouldn't be enjoying the great outdoors, but there are safer ways for our children to do this than we did ourselves.

We know that sunlight damages the skin, and that this leads to premature ageing and sometimes to skin cancer. We also know that formation of moles is linked to sun exposure, and this in turn is linked to the serious skin cancer melanoma. *Damage from the sun starts as soon as you child is exposed to the sun, and accumulates over a lifetime.* The more fair a person is, the more prone they are to this damage. Freckly, red-headed or snowy-haired children with blue eyes are most at risk. Asian and Indian children are more resistant, but can also burn if overexposed to the sun. Children with very dark skins, such as full blood Aboriginals and Africans, rarely burn. This is because pigment in the skin provides natural sun protection. The more you have, the more resistant you are to burning.

A newborn baby has as little pigment in its skin as will ever be there during its life. This is because exposure to sun actually increases the amount of pigment present. It also means that babies are very sensitive to sunlight, and its best to keep them right out of the sun.

Sunlight is most intense in the middle of the day between the hours of 10 a.m. and 2 p.m. (or 11 a.m. and 3 p.m. daylight saving time). This intensity can be increased by being near highly reflective surfaces, such as snow or water. Even though it is less in winter, overexposure in winter can still cause burning.

How much sunlight is too much? It is difficult to be specific about this. Certainly we should all avoid ever getting a sunburn, but even without this the long-term effects of the sun still build up to damage our skins. The aim of sun protection should be to avoid burns completely and to minimise sun exposure without overly compromising our enjoyable lifestyle. Exactly how much this is varies from person to person, and partly depends on the individual's skin type and what are considered to be essential daily activities.

When today's generation of parents were children, sun protection wasn't nearly as well understood as it is today, and modern sunblocks just weren't available. How many of us were told to go out and get a 'healthy tan'? The idea of a tan being equated with health and vigour has been very much part of the Australian mentality, and many still believe that being pale means looking unwell. It is true that we need some sun exposure to form the vitamin D essential for bone health, but you can easily get this from a few minutes in the shade every day. Most of what the sun does to us is damaging, not healthy.

Australian children spend a lot of time outdoors, both at school and on the weekends. It's been estimated that eighty per cent of our lifetime exposure to sun is accumulated before we reach twenty, so this is the time to really concentrate on sun protection.

What is the best way to do this? The first thing to do is simply to avoid the sun. Try to stay indoors or in the shade during the middle of the day. If you do go out then, use protective clothes and sunscreens. If you are driving, keep the windows closed if you can. Glass screens out a lot of harmful rays.

As far as clothing goes, dark coloured close-weave clothes give the best protection. Although light clothing can be relatively transparent to sunlight, for the most part clothing gives very good sun protection. Try to dress your child in clothes that cover as much of the skin as possible, without being too hot. Choose all-in-one swimsuits which cover the trunk, or include a swim shirt. Fortunately these items can be highly fashionable! Include in your child's outfit a wide-brimmed or flap hat, and if possible a pair of sunglasses as we know that sun also damages the eyes.

Even with protective clothing there are some areas of skin, such as the face and lower arms and hands, that just don't get covered up, and these need the help of a sunscreen. Adult Australians always show the most sun damage in these areas, and this is because they are always exposed to light.

Sunscreens work because they contain chemicals which absorb ultraviolet (UV) light as well as reflecting substances which bounce it off the skin. They should be rated with an **SPF** (sun protection factor) **number**. What this number means is how long you can stay outside without burning when using the sunscreen. If you can stay out in midday sun for 10 minutes before you just start to burn, a sunscreen with an SPF rating of 15 will give you fifteen times ten minutes in the sun, or two and a half hours, on any one day. You can't increase this by reapplying the sunscreen, or by putting on two layers of it, but if you add to this being in the shade you'll get a lot more time outdoors without burning. Sweating heavily and swimming can diminish the time you get from your sunscreen, so if this happens, re-apply it. When putting on sunscreen don't skimp, and make sure that all exposed areas are covered well. Allow about thirty minutes between applying the cream and going out in the sun, as it takes about this long to reach maximum effectiveness. And check the expiry date on the bottle to make sure the product is still effective. If it has expired, you're probably not using enough!

Sunscreens come in a bewildering array. There are creams, gels, lotions and sprays, sticks for your lips and around your eyes. They can be found in moisturisers and makeups, and in a very wide range of prices. In general it is true to say that the inexpensive ones are as good as the expensive ones, as long as the SPF is clearly stated. Beware of any sunscreen without a stated SPF, and always choose the highest rating you can get. There is no point buying something which will give you only half an hour in the sun before you burn. Your choice of sunscreen is a personal one, depending on what you find most pleasant to use.

Parents often ask if sunscreens are safe, especially on babies. They worry about the protective chemicals in sunscreens, and wonder if they are just as dangerous in the long term as getting burnt. It is true that it is possible to be allergic to the chemicals, and sometimes to the perfume or preservatives in sunscreens, and this can produce a rash. Although this is itchy it isn't dangerous and will resolve when the sunscreen is stopped. Sometimes, sunscreens can cause stinging, especially if they get into the eyes. Again this isn't dangerous, but means that your child is sensitive to the protective chemicals. And of course, once a child has had this experience it can be difficult to get them to co-operate with having sunscreen put on their faces ever again!

As far as we know, sunscreens are safe, and don't cause cancer. Compare this to everything we know about the potential of sunlight to cause cancer, and it would appear that sunscreens are definitely the lesser of the two evils. In addition, consider that other things we put on our skins every day without a moment's thought, such as makeup, or perfumes, are also 'chemicals'. If you just can't get this concern out of your mind, however, there are more and more sunscreens coming on the market which are 'chemical free'. They rely on the inert substances, titanium and zinc, to reflect light away from the skin. Because they do not contain the UV-protective chemicals, they don't tend to sting sensitive eyes and are suitable for children who are allergic to other sunscreens. They often don't have quite as high an SPF as sunscreens containing chemicals that absorb ultraviolet light, but if the alternative is no sunscreen at all because of concern about synthetic chemicals, then they are a very good alternative. But if your child is going boating, or skiing in the middle of the day, or standing out in the sun playing cricket, please drop your concerns and get the strongest sunblock you can, even if it's just once in a while. Ask you chemist about the most effective ones, as it can be very hard to know what they are unless you know what all the names in the formulation really mean. In addition, extra block in the form of zinc, for example the fluorescent zinc sticks now available, can give worthwhile extra protection for lips, noses and cheeks. These areas seem to be the most prone to sunburn on the face.

Having said all this, no one would suggest that we all start to live like hermits. It is just not practical to expect children to remain inside all day, or not to go to the pool or the beach, or not to play sports outdoors. However it's sensible to put as many sun-protection techniques into their lives as possible from the first time they get exposed to sun, and this should be all year round, not just in summer. In school, too, sun protection should be a part of the routine. Check if your school has a sun protection policy, and if they don't, do something about it! Eventually you may even find that your children are reminding you about sun protection. When you get them to this point, you have really achieved something!

Australian children will probably always get more sun than their counterparts in cold climates, and, being realistic, Australians will probably always be more damaged by the sun than many others, but our attitudes and sun avoidance habits are certainly improving. Let's hope this generation has much less of a problem in adult life as a result of sun damage than the ones before it.

NITS AND OTHER INSECTS

Nits (head lice)

Very few children go through childhood without an attack of head lice. These creatures are tiny creatures known as mites, and are so small that you need a microscope to see them properly. They live on the scalp and lay their eggs on hairs.

These eggs, the 'nits', are easily seen as egg-shaped white specks, firmly attached to the hair. The scalp becomes itchy, and often little red bites can be seen on the nape of the neck.

Head lice are very contagious. It's not uncommon for many children at a school to be infected, as the mite is easily transmitted from one child to the other.

Fortunately, head lice are easily recognised and treated. Your chemist can show you a variety of shampoos to use. It's most important, however, that absolutely everyone in the families of all the affected children be treated, and that the treatment be done on two occasions a week apart. In addition, combs, brushes, hats and whatever goes on your head should be washed. If these precautions aren't taken you run the risk of getting reinfected after you have done the treatment.

Scabies

This is another highly contagious infection with a small mite. It is less common than head lice, and a lot more difficult to recognise in many cases.

Scabies can only be caught from other human beings. It cannot be acquired from any other type of animal. When the mite gets onto the skin, it makes a small curved, scaly burrow in the surface where it lives. These are usually found on the hands and in between the fingers. In babies, these burrows are found on the palms and soles and often cause little blisters. The mite lays its eggs in the burrow, and soon after dies. The eggs hatch and the whole thing starts over again.

There may be only a few mites on a child's body, living in their burrows, but their presence sets up an allergic reaction which causes widespread itching and a rash. Often children also have red lumps under their arms and around the groin. Eventually other members of the family become infected and start to itch, although the extent to which each person is affected varies, and some may seem to have no symptoms at all.

The mention of the word scabies tends to make people feel a bit unclean, as though they have acquired it from lack of hygiene. As a result, they sometimes deny that they could possibly have it, thus delaying treatment while they infect more people. In fact, scabies is just an infection like any other, and if you catch it why feel ashamed? All it means is that you have made close contact with someone else who has it, exactly the same as catching a cold.

Treating scabies follows the same principles as treating head lice but it is somewhat more difficult. A cream containing an appropriate insecticide, which can be obtained over the counter from the chemist, should be applied to the affected people and everyone in their household. Other people who should be treated include children whom your child plays with regularly and their families, baby sitters, day care minders and any relatives who mind the children. Sometimes the list can run to dozens of people, especially in big families. Treating everyone can be quite an undertaking and can become quite expensive as well, but if it isn't done properly, like nits, the infection just goes round and round.

There are two insecticide creams available which skin specialists usually recommend. One contains a substance called lindane, the other is called permethrin. People are often worried about the safety of putting these on their children, as they are synthetic chemicals, but both appear to be very safe, and cause little trouble other than some dryness and temporary irritation after they have been applied. Lindane has been around for many years and has stood the test of time. Permethrin has recently become available in Australia.

When applying the creams make sure that they are put absolutely everywhere on the skin from the neck down, and under the nails. In babies the scalp should be treated too. If the hands are washed during the day, the cream should be reapplied to them. A minimum of eight hours is recommended for leaving the cream on, but sometimes this may be inadequate and as much as 48 hours is required.

If you are using lindane, it has to be reapplied in the same way one week later. Permethrin only needs to be used once.

It is very important that at the end of your treatment you wash all the clothes, towels and sheets that you have used in the last two weeks. You don't have to fumigate the furniture. This is because your skin doesn't make direct contact with it, unless of course you are in the habit of sitting on it with no clothes on! If you have items that make contact with your skin which you just can't wash, such as woolly slippers, put them away for a couple of weeks. If there are any mites on them, they'll die if they can't get back onto your skin.

If all this is done properly scabies is easy to clear up, so don't panic if you are diagnosed as having it. And remember, it can happen to anyone!

Other insects

There are lots of other insects which can bite children. Mosquitoes, fleas and paspalum mites are the ones which cause the most trouble. None of us would have much trouble in identifying an insect bite if we saw one. Trouble can start however if you have a child who is very allergic to bites.

Some children are really sensitive to insect bites. It starts when they are around two and may last a few years before a tolerance develops. Whenever such a child is bitten they come up in big itchy lumps and sometimes blisters which can then become infected. These bites are nearly always on the arms, legs and face, as these are the parts of the skin accessible to the insects. Every time the child gets bitten, it can reactivate all the other recent bites, so they can easily end up covered with lumps and blisters.

Fortunately insect problems are seasonal in temperate regions, happening mainly in spring and summer, with recovery occurring in winter and autumn. In tropical areas, however, the problem may last all year.

How do you deal with an insect bite problem in your child? The first thing to do is deal with the insects. Mosquitoes, being airborne, are best kept out with screens. Avoiding being outside at night and avoiding having stagnant water, in which they breed, near the house, is also important. Fleas live on pets, in sandpits and on carpets and furniture, so getting rid of them involves treating the pets and fumigating the house. Paspalum mites are a seasonal problem, and live in long paspalum grass. Keeping this short is the answer here.

The second thing to do is protect your child. Long pants are a good idea when playing outside, as most insect bites occur on the legs, but this isn't always practical in summer. Insect repellents are helpful, and if you are worried about the safety of them on your child's skin, spray them onto their clothes.

As far as treating an established bite goes, there is little you can do other than apply calamine lotion to relieve the itch. Cortisone creams can be useful, but only partially so, and if there is a lot of swelling antihistamines can help. However once a bite has happened, you really just have to wait for it to settle down, which in a very allergic child can take as long as two weeks. So when it comes to insect bites and children, prevention is definitely better than cure.

ALLERGIC SKIN PROBLEMS IN CHILDREN

Apart from allergy to insect bites, there are a couple of other common allergic skin rashes that occur in children. One is allergy to plants, and the other is hives, also known as urticaria.

Allergy to plants

Plant allergy occurs when a child's bare skin makes contact with a plant to which he or she is allergic. The contact with the plant can be very brief, lasting only seconds, and often happens when the child runs past a bush which brushes against the skin. Shortly afterwards, usually starting after a couple of hours, the skin becomes itchy, and red, blistery streaks appear, corresponding to the areas touched by the plant. This worsens gradually over the next few days, with patches coming up all over the place—anywhere the plant touched. If untreated the problem can take two weeks or more to settle.

Many plants can cause this kind of allergy, but there are only a couple which very commonly do this. One is the *rhus* tree, and the other is the *grevillea* bush, most often the very popular grevillea 'Robyn Gordon' which is planted in so many parks and school playgrounds.

Adults are just as prone to this type of allergy, which we call contact allergy because it is the result of contact of an allergy-causing substance (the *allergen*) with the skin. However adults often develop this as a result of contact with medications, cosmetics, perfumes and industrial chemicals—things that children don't come into contact with. Adults, on the other hand, don't tend to go running or rolling through the bushes in their swimming costumes, nor do they usually climb trees. This is why plants are the commonest cause of contact allergy in children.

A severe attack of plant allergy usually requires treatment with cortisone, and this needs to be carefully supervised by your doctor.

Hives (urticaria)

Hives are very common. It has been estimated that at least one in ten people get an attack at some time in their lives. If this has ever happened to you, then you know all about it.

Hives are intensely itchy wheals. They often appear very suddenly, and can occur on any part of the skin. The wheals move about all the time, with new spots appearing while others disappear. Attacks can last anywhere from hours to days.

The rash itself is caused by the release into your skin of a natural chemical called histamine, which is made in your body. Histamine is an important part of your immune system. When people come into contact with an allergy-causing substance (allergen) which produces hives, the immune system goes a little haywire, and releases large amounts of histamine, which is usually only found in traces. The histamine, in excess, causes the itchy, swollen red patches.

Very occasionally, so much histamine can be released that swelling occurs around the eyes, face and throat. This can cause difficulty swallowing and breathing. In very rare instances, the person can collapse and become unconscious. If your child has hives and this seems to be happening, take him straight to hospital—it could save his life.

There are many things which can cause this type of allergic reaction. Foods, medications, insect bites, vaccinations and pollens can all do it. These are things that are swallowed, injected or inhaled. Another common cause of hives in children is a simple viral illness. The duration of the attack is related to how long it takes for the allergy-causing substance to be eradicated from your system. This is why length of attacks is so variable, and in the case of viruses, can last a few weeks. It's not at all uncommon for a child to be allergic to some common substance which is being eaten every day, and in such cases the hives can seem to be continuous for many weeks.

If your child has hives, the attacks can usually be relieved with antihistamines, which can be obtained from the chemist. But make sure you know what the skin rash is before you treat it. This may require a visit to your doctor. Fortunately most attacks are brief, and only when the problem becomes long-standing will your child need investigation to determine the cause of the allergy. Be patient, and in most cases the attack will be over in a week or two. Remember that although hives are itchy and uncomfortable, it is almost always a harmless allergic condition.

SOME COMMON SKIN INFECTIONS YOU SHOULD KNOW ABOUT

Impetigo (school sores)

Impetigo is an infection with a germ called golden staph. This is the commonest cause of skin infections of all kinds, and the most frequent of these in children is impetigo. Many people have heard of golden staph and associate it with serious infection. This can certainly be the case, but it just as often causes relatively harmless skin problems.

Impetigo is highly infectious, and is usually caught from other children. It often involves several members of a family at once. It can be recognised as crusty or scabby sores which have a yellowish look about them. They are not as a rule terribly painful but can be itchy. Sometimes impetigo causes big blisters, particularly in babies. The commonest sites for the sores are the face and around the groin area, but they can occur anywhere.

It's not unusual for impetigo to occur when there is another skin problem present, such as head lice, scabies or eczema.

Treatment of impetigo involves using antibiotics, which must be obtained on prescription from your doctor. These can be given in either oral or ointment form, depending on the severity of the problem.

Usually clearing up impetigo is no problem at all, but in some cases the golden staph can really get to like you, and live persistently on your skin. This results in the problem recurring almost as soon as it has been treated. Such cases may require several weeks of disinfection, not only of the child involved, but the whole family as well, as more often than not other members will also be infected. If this is happening to your child, you should see your doctor.

Ringworm (tinea)

Ringworm is not a worm, it is a fungal infection. It isn't quite as infectious as golden staph. It can be acquired from other people, but children often catch it from the family pet. A new kitten or guinea pig is often the culprit.

On the skin, ringworm usually forms a characteristic circular rash, hence its name. The edge of the ring is red and scaly, and it spreads out, leaving patches of normal skin in the centre. It's usually quite itchy. If not treated, it may last for many weeks or months.

In children, ringworm can also affect the scalp. This is very rare in adults, who have greasy scalps which are inhospitable to the infection. As a result of ringworm of the scalp, bald patches appear. They are itchy and scaly, and contain brittle, easily pulled out, or broken-off hairs. Sometimes the scalp is not scaly at all but the hairs break off close to the scalp, leaving black dots. There are usually several bald patches present.

In adults, the commonest spots for tinea ('athlete's foot') are the feet and groin, and other people, rather than pets, are the source. In children this is uncommon, although teenagers may suffer from the same sorts of infections as adults.

Fungal infections are usually easy to recognise and treat. For uncomplicated infections on the skin, treatment with antifungal creams, many of which are available from the chemist, is usually successful, provided they are used regularly every day for at least three weeks. However if the infection is on the scalp, it is essential to use oral medication, and this usually takes a minimum of six to twelve weeks of treatment. You must see your doctor about this.

Cold sores (Herpes simplex)

Cold sores are another very common skin infection. They are caused by a virus called herpes simplex. The mention of herpes usually raises a lot of anxiety, as most people associate this name with a sexually transmitted disease. Indeed the cold sore virus is related to the one that causes genital herpes, but it has a very different mode of infection.

The cold sore infection is probably acquired by most people at some time in childhood. It is so widespread that it is practically impossible *not* to be exposed to it. Some people seem to have a natural resistance, while others suffer from severe attacks. It all depends on the way you're made.

The first attack of cold sores can be quite severe, and can cause a very painful ulcerated mouth, associated with an unpleasant illness which makes the child quite unwell. After this the body's immune system holds the virus in check, but seems never to be able to get rid of it completely. As a result, minor attacks recur at irregular intervals, usually when the child has a cold, or gets sunburnt or has other illnesses. Usually, with time, these attacks get less frequent and severe, but cold sores can keep recurring all through life. This is a nuisance, but is not dangerous.

The usual place for cold sores is on the lips, but they can occur on other parts of the face, and rarely on the rest of the skin. The sore itself is preceded by a tingly feeling, and soon after a group of clear blisters appear, which quickly form a scab, healing after about a week.

Once a cold sore has formed, there is little that can be done to stop it progressing, or speed up healing. Various cold sore remedies are sold by the chemist. What these do is minimise the symptoms of the cold sore, but they don't stop the natural progression. If cold sores become a really severe problem, and fortunately this is rare, see your doctor, as preventative treatment is available.

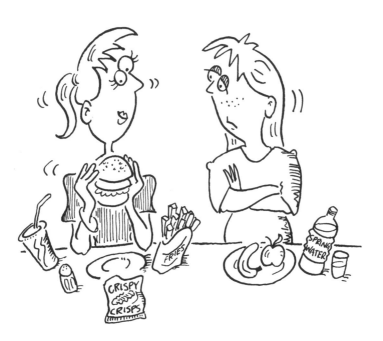

CHAPTER TWO

A SPOT OF BOTHER

Skin problems in adolescence

ANNETTE CALLAN

THE ROLE OF HORMONES

When it comes to certain skin problems, women are at the mercy of their hormones. A hormone is a 'chemical messenger', made in a gland called an **endocrine** gland. From there it is carried in the bloodstream to the various tissues of the body where it influences growth and how the tissue functions. Before a hormone can affect the target tissue, the cells in this tissue must contain a specific receptor for that hormone, into which it fits like a key into a lock.

Our skin is a target for sex hormones. Many of the blemishes and cosmetically annoying problems which concern women, such as excess facial and body hair, oily skin and acne, are greatly influenced by sex hormones.

The smooth unblemished facial skin of the prepubertal 8- or 9-year-old girl becomes open-pored, oily and acne-prone in the 12-13 year old. Blackheads start to appear on the chin and nose, the skin and scalp become increasingly oily, and downy hair appears on the upper lip. These changes are largely brought about by **androgens**, so-called 'male' sex hormones. From puberty to menopause, a woman's ovaries, which are endocrine glands as well as sources of ova (eggs), produce androgens as well as the female sex hormones oestrogen and progesterone. Women also form androgens in other endocrine glands situated just above the kidneys—the adrenal glands. So it is not strictly accurate to refer to androgens as 'male' hormones. Androgens vary in strength, and some parts of our skin have the capacity to convert weak androgens into stronger ones so that the net effect on a woman's skin may be significant. A woman does not produce nearly as much androgen as an adult male.

In our skin the hair follicles and the oil producing glands (**sebaceous glands**) exist as a combined structure called the **pilo-sebaceous unit** (pilus is Latin for 'hair', sebum means 'grease'). Sebum is the oily substance which lubricates the surface of human skin and hair. The sebaceous gland discharges sebum (oil) into the same canal or duct through which the hair emerges from the skin, this common channel being referred to as the **pilo-sebaceous duct**. (See diagram 1.)

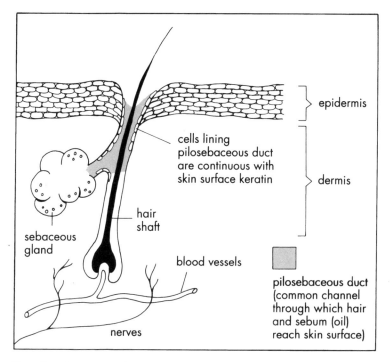

The pilo-sebaceous unit

In some areas of skin, such as the nose and T-zone of the face, the sebaceous glands are very large in comparison to their associated hair follicles.

It is the pilo-sebaceous units in certain areas of our skin which are targets for androgens. They are 'primed' to respond to androgen stimulation, especially those on the face, centre of the chest and upper back. Hair follicles in the midline areas of the body, which roughly correspond to the pattern of male body and facial hair, are highly androgen-sensitive. So also is the top of the scalp where, paradoxically, androgens cause *diminished* rather than *increased* hair growth, resulting in typical male balding. (See chapter 4.)

Puberty

In childhood the sebaceous glands produce only small amounts of sebum. Body hair is fine and lightly pigmented, except for that on the scalp, eyebrows and eyelashes. Around the age of 9 to 11 androgens start being formed in the adrenal glands. These hormones are responsible for the earliest signs of adult sexual development, namely the gradual appearance of coarse pubic and underarm hair. It is at this time that sebaceous glands in certain body areas grow larger and produce significantly more sebum—hence the formation of 'open pores' and blackheads on the nose and chin and noticeably oilier skin and scalp.

This becomes more pronounced as the ovaries commence their rhythmic cycles of hormone and egg production with the onset of menstrual periods around age 12 to 14. Once the sebaceous glands begin to function at an adult level the stage is set for the development of problem oily skin and acne—and unwanted hair growth on the face and body.

ACNE IN YOUNG WOMEN

Pimples, or 'zits', or **acne vulgaris,** are very common during adolescence. Almost every young person experiences them to some degree.

Genetic predisposition largely determines whether or not acne occurs and how severe it will be. For example, severe cystic acne, which consists of large swellings and pus-filled cysts that eventually heal with unpleasant scarring, tends to run in some families and affects about 5 per cent of the population. Cystic acne and other severe types of acne can be emotionally devastating for young people growing into adulthood in a society which places so much emphasis on an attractive physical appearance.

Causes of acne—what we know

Dermatologists recognise that acne is an extremely complex condition with a number of causes.

The androgen hormones which first appear in significant amounts around puberty stimulate immature sebaceous glands to become fully functional adult glands in certain areas of skin. Stimulation by androgens is a *pre-requisite* for the development of acne. Males castrated before puberty (eunuchs) do not develop oily skin, blackheads or acne in later life. No androgens, no acne! Hormonal factors create the scenario in which acne develops. *Over-production of sebum* (oil) is regarded as *one* of the causes of acne.

But this is not the full story. *Blockage of the pilo-sebaceous duct*, the small canal which connects the sebaceous gland to the skin surface, seems to be the starting point for the acne pimple. Here the cells lining the duct and around its opening to the skin surface clump together and form a plug which results in a blackhead. (A blackhead consists of dead skin cells and dried sebum filling a dilated sebaceous duct. The black colour is from the effect of air on the surface of the plug; a whitehead is essentially the same but without an opening to the surface.) Minute blackheads, not visible to the naked eye, occur in acne-prone skin and are often the starting point for acne pimples.

Below the blockage of the sebaceous duct, *bacteria* multiply, producing chemical substances which react with the accumulated dead cells and stagnant sebum. This causes *inflammation* in the sebaceous gland and surrounding tissue, leading to a pimple. Acne is never contagious and it is not an infection in the strict sense of the word. The bacteria involved are usually harmless and are normal inhabitants of large oil ducts in all healthy adults. They only become a problem in blocked, over-active sebaceous glands. White cells from the blood stream gather in the area of inflammation around the blocked sebaceous gland, and if there are large numbers of these, a pus-filled pimple ensues. If a number of adjoining sebaceous glands are simultaneously affected, large acne cysts develop. The amount of scarring left as healing occurs depends on how deep-seated and extensive the inflammation is.

So acne is caused by a combination of things:

- overactive sebaceous glands
- blockage of sebaceous ducts
- bacterial activity
- inflammation in the surrounding tissues.

Acne myths

Acne is not due to greasy food, excessive carbohydrate in the diet, chocolate, nuts or dairy foods; nor will drinking copious amounts of water help. There is no scientific evidence that diet has any influence on acne whatsoever, which may come as a surprise to people who are convinced that chocolate causes 'breakouts'. Long hair and greasy fringes falling forward over the face and forehead do not make acne worse. Sometimes the hair style is a deliberate ploy by the acne sufferer to help hide the affected skin.

Acne has nothing to do with lack of cleanliness. This common misconception probably comes about because the black substance of blackheads is mistaken for dirt. Acne does not magically clear on your 21st birthday, nor necessarily vanish after the first baby. Some women develop acne for the first time after the age of 20, and a significant number still have acne in the late 20s and early 30s. Acne often improves in pregnancy, but in some women it occurs for the first time or worsens during pregnancy.

Sun exposure is not a good acne treatment. What actually happens is that a tan camouflages pimples to some degree. In addition, the accelerated shedding of skin surface cells which follows sunburn may temporarily alleviate sebaceous duct blockages. This process of 'exfoliation' (or inducing a mild peel) is actually the basis of some external treatments used in acne. But the benefits are short-lived, and should be weighed against the potential long term harmful effects of ultraviolet exposure (see chapter 8). Self-treatment with sun lamps is not advised in the light of what we know about the causes of skin cancer and photoageing.

It is a myth that deep cleansing facials will help acne. The completely illogical suggestion that pores, which are in reality the openings of pilo-sebaceous ducts, can be 'opened up' and cleansed deep down to remove 'impurities' is a myth. It is true that blackheads can be expressed and that pre-steaming may facilitate this by softening the keratin around the plugged duct opening, but blackheads will reform within days, and unless other treatments are used to reduce blackhead formation, there will be no net benefit. Pores cannot be closed or tightened with 'toners' or 'astringents', nor can any other applied cream stimulate sluggish circulation and remove 'toxic waste'. Acne masks and astringents have a mildly irritant action on skin, causing a minute degree of swelling around sebaceous pores and thus making them temporarily less conspicuous. Some of these agents are also degreasing and help temporarily make the skin *feel* less oily. Washing with soap and water will achieve the same result.

What makes acne worse?

Stress does not cause acne but if you have acne, stress may worsen it. Whilst we do not know exactly how this happens, we do know that certain androgen hormones made by the adrenal gland increase in the bloodstream during stressful periods. Having acne can be a *source* of stress for many women, leading to lack of confidence and poor self-esteem.

Heat and humidity can worsen acne, probably because sweating aggravates the pore blockages by increasing the water content of the outermost skin layers. *Oily cosmetics* can aggravate acne by increasing pore obstruction and blackhead formation. People working in an oily industry where cutting oils and greases contact the skin sometimes develop acne in unusual areas, such as on the thighs due to contact with oil-soaked overalls. Similarly massage oils may promote acne. *Some medications* aggravate acne or cause acne-like skin eruptions. Such drugs include steroids and drugs related to androgens, particularly anabolic steroids taken by some athletes. Other drugs, including lithium and some anti-epilepsy drugs, can also occasionally aggravate acne or cause an acne-like rash. *Squeezing* and *picking* acne spots can undoubtedly worsen the situation by increasing inflammation. The result is a longer-lasting pimple and sometimes damage to the surrounding tissues and hence permanent scarring.

How long does acne last in women?

Although the earliest signs of acne may be visible at age 8 or 9, outbreaks are rare under the age of 10. Girls tend to develop acne earlier than boys since they reach puberty earlier. It is estimated that about 40 per cent of girls aged 14–17 have acne.

The overwhelming tendency is for acne to steadily decrease with age. Some cases resolve without scarring in only a few months, others smoulder for years. Sometimes breakouts are interspersed with acne-free periods. Some women may have a relatively acne-free adolescence only to develop significant problems in their twenties. Around 5 per cent of women still suffer from acne at age 40.

Acne treatment

Acne should never be dismissed as a trivial complaint which the sufferer will eventually 'grow out of'. Acne can be both disfiguring and embarrassing, and scarring resulting from severe acne can leave its mark on the psyche as well as on the skin.

Treatment of acne must be tailored to the individual sufferer. Dermatologists are guided by the severity and type of acne, areas affected, age of patient, family history, and whether or not a patient has any other medical problems. Pregnant and breast-feeding women have special requirements. Cystic acne needs more potent forms of treatment than other types of acne. A pre-pubertal girl with mainly blackheads and whiteheads and relatively few inflamed pimples will need a different approach from a woman nearing menopause. The personal preferences of the individual patient will also be taken into account. Treatment programs are aimed at one or more of the main causes, namely the over-production of sebum, blockage of sebaceous ducts, bacterial activity, and inflammation.

Cleaning the skin in acne

Washing is important to remove grime and surface oil, make-up and dead surface cells. Ideally this should be done twice daily with a mild soap and water or a non-oily soap substitute. The proverbial 'good scrub' will only irritate the skin. Abrasive cleansers, cleansing granules and abrasive sponges are not generally recommended. Because there is always a background of overproduction of oil in acne, most external applications prescribed are in the form of non-oily or alcohol-based lotions or gels which tend to dry the skin. If, in addition, the skin is over-washed or scrubbed excessively the result is uncomfortable flakiness.

Anti-bacterial soaps are not necessary because the bacteria involved are part of the skin's normal 'flora' and are furthermore located deep in the oil ducts where soap will have little effect. These types of cleansing agents are generally too irritating. Sometimes it is appropriate to use special cleansing agents, for example those containing a weak mixture of salicylic acid, which encourages shedding of surface cells by producing a mild peel. Other cleansing agents contain benzoyl peroxide, which counteracts acne by penetrating the follicle and reducing bacterial activity as well as causing a mild peeling effect. These types of cleansers might be introduced to supplement mild soap and water washing in a treatment program. Because soaps and cleansing agents are rinsed off immediately after being applied, they can only have a limited therapeutic effect as their contact time with the skin is so short.

Externally applied acne treatment (topical applications)

In the past **sulfur, salicylic acid** and **resorcinol** were the main ingredients of acne applications. These chemicals help by producing a mild peel and/or having a mild anti-bacterial effect. Although they are still used they have been largely superseded by more effective products. Some sulfur-containing applications can be useful as they come as flesh tinted creams which can be used as a make-up substitute to camouflage blemishes. The mild peel caused by salicylic acid helps unclog pores and loosen blackheads and, when combined with alcohol in a lotion form, it helps temporarily degrease the surface. The peeling and flaking produced by these applications will not suit everybody. Some people with problem oily skin may find them quite useful.

Benzoyl peroxide is particularly useful with its two-pronged attack on bacteria and clogged pores. It is available

as alcohol- or water-based gels, masks and washes in varying strengths. It is usually advisable to start with the weakest
(2.5%) and gradually move up to 5% or even 10% as your
skin gradually becomes tolerant. Oily skin may be able to
tolerate the alcohol-based gel, whereas more sensitive or
more mature skin is best treated with the water-based preparations. Benzoyl peroxide can bleach clothing and bed linen,
which some people find annoying. Very rarely some people
develop an allergy to benzoyl peroxide that makes its use
impossible.

Azaleic acid in a topical cream works by reducing blackheads, decreasing bacterial activity and reducing inflammation and may cause less peeling and irritation than benzoyl
peroxide. It may take several weeks before an effect is
noticed.

Tretinoin is a topical treatment particularly aimed at dis-
lodging blackheads by its effect on the keratin lining the oil
ducts. It is available as gel, cream and lotion. Tretinoin
should not be used in pregnancy or when breast feeding.
People using topical tretinoin usually experience some redness and flaking initially. Sometimes the acne pimples appear
more inflamed in the first six weeks until the skin builds up
a tolerance. If persevered with, the inflammation will eventually reduce as the sebaceous ducts become unblocked.
Tretinoin is also a potential sun sensitiser so that you will
sunburn more easily on areas where it has been applied. This
should not detract from its use, as non-oily sunscreens can
be used in conjunction. More recently, **isotretinoin** has
become available as a topical application. It has the same
effect as topical tretinoin but with less irritation.

Antibiotic lotions are useful in combating the bacterial
side of acne. They can be formulated in alcoholic bases, or
as non-oily lotions if alcohol is too drying for your skin.
Although they are usually not as effective, they can be useful
in patients who cannot or prefer not to use antibiotics by
mouth. Dermatologists often combine these antibiotic
lotions with other topical treatments.

How should acne applications be used?

Topical treatments should be applied to clean skin. If the skin is moist the irritant effect of topicals will be enhanced so it is probably best, if possible, to wait ten or fifteen minutes after washing before applying your lotions or gels, or to ensure at least that you have dried your skin thoroughly. It is certainly advisable to wait about ten minutes after washing before applying tretinoin. It is also advisable to apply it at least half an hour before going to bed to minimise spreading to the corners of the mouth and eyelids, which are more easily irritated. Bed-time is usually a good time to apply any topical treatment designed to be used only once daily. It is also the best time to apply tretinoin because of its sun sensitising potential. Most topical preparations are not highly visible on the skin, so can be worn during the day and applied under make-up.

Make-up and moisturisers in acne

Most young acne suffers have excessively oily skin, making the routine use of moisturisers unnecessary. Dryness and irritation should not be a problem if you start with lower strengths of topicals and build up to greater strengths, allowing the skin to adjust gradually. Sometimes alternate-day treatments are appropriate if your skin is very sensitive.

Unfortunately, when dryness and irritation from topical treatments become a problem, some women undo all the good work by using the wrong types of moisturiser. Oily moisturisers only aggravate acne by clogging pores and encouraging blackhead formation. Oil-free moisturisers can be used if dry skin becomes a problem. Likewise oil-free foundations should be used. Excellent oil-free make-ups are available which are suitable for acne patients and give good matt coverage.

Loose and compact pressed powder don't make acne worse. For people wishing to camouflage particularly noticeable spots, oil-free cover sticks and flesh-tinted acne creams containing sulfur are available.

Sunscreens for acne

Sunscreens for acne-affected areas should also be oil-free. Alcohol-based products are completely oil-free but tend to sting (especially when reapplied throughout the day). Some lotions and creams are also suitable, but you should avoid thick greasy products as they encourage pore clogging.

Antibiotic treatment of acne

Antibiotics suppress the more severe types of acne. There are no hard and fast rules as to how long treatment should be continued. In general, if a person's acne is sufficiently severe to warrant oral antibiotic treatment, a six-month course would be a minimum treatment time. The most commonly prescribed antibiotics are **tetracyclines**. These drugs have few side effects or disadvantages. **Erythromycin** and **sulphonamide** antibiotics are sometimes used, for example in people who are unable to take tetracyclines for various reasons. The aim is to treat with antibiotics until the acne is adequately suppressed and then gradually to decrease the dose to a maintenance level, finally ceasing altogether once the acne clears satisfactorily. Two to three months' treatment at the higher doses may be needed before a definite improvement is noticed.

Antibiotics wipe out some of the bacteria in sebaceous ducts, reducing their chemical action on the lipids (fats) in sebum. They also have an anti-inflammatory action. The choice of antibiotic, dosage and duration of treatment is a matter of fine tuning. Some patients respond rapidly, others less so and some may require prolonged or repeated courses. It all depends on age, genetic predisposition, skin type and severity of acne—the factors which your dermatologist will take into account before deciding on the type and dosage of antibiotic.

Patients sometimes ask if there is any point in using a treatment which is only suppressive and not a guaranteed 'cure'. The answer is a definite yes. Prompt and adequate antibiotic treatment may convert a severe acne into a more manageable, milder type. Reduced inflammation and fewer pimples mean less scarring.

*When should you **not** take antibiotics?*

Tetracycline antibiotics should not be taken in pregnancy or while breast feeding or by children under twelve. They are known to adversely affect development of an unborn child, the danger period being around ten to twelve weeks into the pregnancy. They also cause discolouration of developing teeth so should not be taken until the permanent teeth are through. Erythromycin is safe in pregnancy and pre-adolescence.

Some tetracyclines must be taken on an empty stomach (half to one hour before a meal or two hours after) and should not be taken with milk or iron tablets, both of which decrease drug absorption and lessen their effect.

Side effects of tetracyclines

Tetracycline antibiotics are extremely safe provided the precautions outlined above are taken. Allergic reactions are rare and take the form of rashes often like hives or measles. Some patients say that they are 'allergic' to a particular medication when what they really mean is that the drug has caused nausea or stomach irritation. This is not true allergy, and mostly can be avoided by using one of the tetracyclines which may be taken with food. Unfortunately there is no scientific way to predict whether one is going to become allergic to a prescribed medication like tetracycline or, for that matter, any other medication.

Antibiotics like tetracycline are known as 'broad spectrum'. This means that they are effective against a wide range of bacteria. A spin-off from this totally desirable effect in acne is that these drugs may reduce the number of certain bacteria in the bowel and the vagina which constitute the normal 'flora' in these areas. (See chapter 5.) This may allow an increase in the growth of another member of the normal flora, a yeast called candida, resulting in vaginal thrush. Although this can be trying for some women, it is treatable and does not affect general health.

Tetracyclines and some other antibiotics may reduce the effectiveness of oral contraceptives by causing a drop in the blood level of oestrogen. Women taking the Pill for birth control must be warned of this possibility and be prepared to use additional contraceptive measures when on this combination, particularly in the first few months of taking the combination.

Ro-accutane (oral isotretinoin)

This medication is designed for cystic acne and severe acne, the cases which fail to respond to the more conventional treatment. It is truly one of the modern wonder drugs, since it cures acne in around 80–90 per cent of cases and permanently and dramatically improves the remainder.

Ro-Accutane is a synthetic drug based on Vitamin A which targets three of the main problems in acne. It decreases the sebaceous gland function so effectively that for a while the sebaceous glands revert to pre-pubertal levels of oil production. It decreases blockage of sebaceous ducts by reducing the keratin build-up. It also has an anti-inflammatory action. A minimum course of around five or six months is needed.

Ro-Accutane has some troublesome side effects, such as dry lips, dry skin, and dry lining of the nose. Minor nose bleeds can be a problem. It is also a photosensitiser, which means that it causes the skin to be more sensitive to ultraviolet rays and thus to sunburn more easily. Oil-free sunscreens should to be used whenever there is a likelihood of sun exposure. Occasionally mild joint pains, mild backache, headaches and tiredness can be a problem. All these side effects can be dealt with effectively as they arise and all disappear quickly once the treatment is stopped.

One of the most important aspects of Ro-Accutane treatment is the need for regular monitoring, around monthly, by the treating dermatologist. Blood tests are necessary before commencing treatment, mainly to ensure that the liver is healthy (since the drug is broken down by the liver), and that the patient does not suffer from high cholesterol levels (since in some patients Ro-Accutane causes a temporary rise in cholesterol and triglyceride in the bloodstream).

A pregnancy test is usually advisable in women before commencing treatment with Ro-Accutane since it must never be taken in pregnancy (or by breast-feeding women) as it can cause birth defects. For this reason, women of child bearing age must be adequately protected against pregnancy and this usually means that oral contraceptives must be taken.

Tackling the hormonal aspects of acne

One way of combating the increase in sebaceous gland activity in women with acne is to take extra oestrogen. Oestrogen helps acne because it increases a protein in the blood known as **sex hormone binding globulin** (SHBG). The function of this protein is to 'soak up' or 'bind' androgens which are floating free in the bloodstream. Only 'free' androgens—not those bound to SHBG—can gain access to the pilo-sebaceous follicles in the skin which are the focus of the acne pimples. Hence the more SHBG in the bloodstream, the more androgen is 'soaked up' by it, with the result that less androgen gets to its target. It is as if the androgen is stuck in a traffic jam of transporter molecules. Incidentally, the high SHBG level in the bloodstream during pregnancy is one of the reasons why acne often tends to clear during pregnancy. Oestrogen is also thought to help acne by directly reducing the activity of the sebaceous gland in some way.

The most convenient way to acquire extra oestrogen is to take an oral contraceptive in which the oestrogen is given cyclically in combination with progestogen. Theoretically, the higher the dose of oestrogen in the birth control pill, the more beneficial for acne. But this also means a higher risk of unwanted side effects, especially the risk of increasing the clotting tendency of the blood. The safest approach is to use a low-dose pill (those containing 35 micrograms of oestrogen) or to take the higher dose (50 micrograms of oestrogen) pill for short periods only.

Most oral contraceptives contain the synthetic progestogen *levonorgestrel*, which has some mild androgen-like effects. It is therefore possible that, in a *minority* of women, the net effect may be a worsening of acne via increased stimulation of oil glands. If this sounds confusing, it at least highlights the fact that no two women metabolise hormones in exactly the same way. It is also an example of how no sex hormone has just one effect. However, because the overall dose of levonorgestrel over the monthly cycle is low, its theoretical adverse effect on acne is probably negligible in most women, and in any case is offset by the beneficial effect of the oestrogen.

Oral contraceptives are available which contain synthetic progestogens that do not have an androgen-like effect and these may be suitable for those women whose acne does not do well with the conventional Pill. **Diane 35ED** has a more dramatic effect in acne. The progestogen in this birth control pill—**cyproterone acetate**—blocks the androgen stimulation of sebaceous glands. In other words, it is an **anti-androgen**. This is the ideal pill for women with acne.

Anti-androgen treatment of acne

Cyproterone acetate in Diane 35ED is an anti-androgen. In other words it blocks the androgen receptor in the pilo-sebaceous follicle, thus preventing androgen from stimulating it. Using the key and lock analogy, an anti-androgen is like a key which fits a lock (the androgen receptor) but will not actually open the door. Cyproterone acetate is taken with oestrogen so is ideal for women who are already taking the Pill. For women unable to take oestrogen or who do not need or want oral contraception, another anti-androgen, **spironolactone**, can be used. Both anti-androgens may be used alone or in combination with antibiotic treatment. Athough anti-androgen treatment suppresses oil production only for as long as it is taken, a course of 6–12 months is often enough to cure or significantly improve acne.

Acne scarring and its treatment

Cosmetically disfiguring acne scarring is the unfortunate outcome of around 7 per cent of acne cases. Different types of scars are seen, including the 'ice-pick' type (punched-out depressions) common on the face, undulating depressed scars, and raised lumpy or cord-like scars which are the sequel of severe cystic acne. Sometimes burnt-out acne cysts may remain as persistent lumps for months or even years. Another common type of scarring which may, paradoxically, follow relatively trivial acne is a white thin scar due to loss of elastic tissue around the affected oil gland. These usually occur on the chest and back in large numbers and look like small white dots. Different types of acne scars may be present in the one patient. Once present, not even Ro-Accutane will eliminate scars, and this is why it is important to treat severe acne early and adequately. Unfortunately, even with adequate treatment, some people are still left with scarring.

A concern for many women are purplish pigmented and sometimes slightly lumpy marks left by burnt-out pimples. These often last for months before eventually fading. They are largely due to excess pigment formation at the site of the pimple and are not true scars since there is no actual destruction of tissue. The lumpiness is due to residual low-grade inflammation and will eventually settle down. Nevertheless, they can be cosmetically annoying as they tend to occur mainly on the face and can be quite noticeable in very fair skin (when they look pink) or very olive skin (when they look purplish/brown).

Techniques used to treat acne scarring include injection with cortisone, dermabrasion and collagen injection. Skin peels can benefit some types of acne scarring and are discussed in chapter 9.

Acne in older women

Dermatologists can't explain why acne doesn't clear with age in some women. In women over 25 whose acne has smouldered on since the teens or who develop acne for the first time, the pimples are often located on the chin, jaw line and neck more than elsewhere on the face. The actual pimples are often firm lumps or 'blind' pimples, and a common complaint is that they tend to linger for many weeks.

Older women with troublesome acne sometimes also have problems with excess hair on the face and/or body, and excessively oily skin. They also frequently notice that the acne becomes more severe before their periods. In some women acne only occurs in the premenstrual week. Only very rarely is mature-age acne due to an 'imbalance' of hormones, that is, over-production of androgens from the ovary or the adrenal glands. Rather, it is due to hypersensitivity of the oil gland to androgens.

When excess production of androgens is suspected appropriate hormone investigations will be ordered by the doctor. Where over-production is discovered, the first aim of treatment is to correct this problem. Otherwise, mature-age acne in women is treated along the same lines as adolescent acne, and in the majority of cases with equally good results. However, because acne in older women seems to be peculiarly sensitive to the effects of androgens, treatment to suppress this hypersensitivity of the oil glands seems to be particularly effective. Cyproterone acetate and Aldactone are both used in this way.

PROBLEM SWEATING

Excessive sweating (doctors call this **hyperhidrosis**) can be distressing for some adolescent girls—affecting the armpits, palms of the hands, soles of the feet, or all three areas. Tell-tale stains on clothing, embarrassing odour and soggy wet palms make social situations an ordeal. In most cases, nervousness or emotional stress are the triggers.

Humans have two types of sweat glands: *apocrine* and *eccrine*. **Apocrine** sweat glands are present in the armpit, in the skin around the nipple, in the genital area and around the anus. Like the sebaceous gland, they are not fully developed until puberty, when they mature under the influence of androgen hormones. Apocrine sweat glands make an oily thick fluid unlike the salty, watery liquid produced by eccrine sweat glands. Bacteria decompose the apocrine sweat and this is what causes the odour which many people prefer to suppress with anti-perspirants and deodorants. Apocrine glands are a relic from a more primitive stage of evolutionary development when body odour played a more important role in human communication. Unpleasant armpit odour can be reduced, not so much by using anti-perspirants and deodorants as by frequent washing. This reduces the number of bacteria and removes stale apocrine sweat before it has a chance to decompose. Antiseptic soaps and antiseptic creams applied at bed-time can also help reduce surface bacteria.

Eccrine sweat glands are present over the whole body surface including the armpits, but are especially numerous on the palms and soles. Eccrine sweating functions as a heat-regulating mechanism in humans to help cool the skin surface by evaporation. Eccrine sweating also occurs in response to mental and emotional stimuli, which is why the palms and soles as well as the armpits become moist when we are nervous, frightened or extremely embarrassed. Whilst eccrine sweat usually has no odour, when it occurs excessively in the armpits it helps to disperse the apocrine sweat, thus leading to increased likelihood of unpleasant odour. Eccrine sweat may also take up the odour of substances like garlic in the diet.

Deodorants contain antiseptics which reduce the skin surface bacteria, thus minimising odour. They usually contain some perfume. Anti-perspirants contain aluminium salts which block eccrine sweat ducts but do not stop apocrine sweat. Perfumes and antiseptic agents are usually included.

Problem underarm perspiration usually needs a stronger preparation than usual. Aluminium chloride hexahydrate 20% in absolute alcohol will usually switch off excess underarm sweating and is available in a number of commercial preparations. It can also be effective on the palms and soles. If this fails, a technique known as **iontophoresis** can be used. This employs a mild electric current to block eccrine sweat ducts and may temporarily inhibit embarrassing sweating.

Medication can be used to block the nerves in the skin that stimulate *eccrine* sweating. Unfortunately it usually causes too many undesirable side effects, such as excessively dry mouth and sometimes disturbances of vision. Extreme excess sweating of the palms and soles that does not respond to other measures can be controlled by surgically cutting the nerves controlling sweating. Unfortunately the resulting dryness may not always be permanent, and there are some dangers associated with this type of operation. Another last resort measure for problem underarm sweating is surgical removal of the area of skin in the armpit that contains the offending sweat glands. Such surgery will, of course, leave the patient with permanent scarring. Fortunately, most cases of excess sweating will eventually resolve without the need for treatment. In most cases it is only a temporary nuisance during adolescence.

CHAPTER THREE

HORMONES ARE A GIRL'S BEST FRIEND

How hormones affect our skin from adolescence to old age

ANNETTE CALLAN

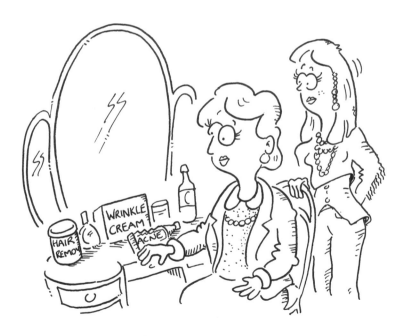

Hormone production continues to change throughout our adult life, and so do the effects on our skin. The changes do not stop with the end of adolescence and pimples.

Problem facial and body hair

In medicine, two terms are used to describe over-abundant hair: *hypertrichosis* and *hirsutism*.

Hirsutism is noticeable growth of coarse, dark hair in those body areas where it is usually regarded as normal for adult males. These typically 'male' areas are the upper lip, cheeks, chin, neck, sideburn area, centre chest, lower abdomen and thighs, buttocks and lower back. Androgen hormones are responsible for the growth of coarse hair in these areas.

In **Hypertrichosis** the excess hair growth is not stimulated by androgens and tends to be finer and lighter than in hirsutism. Hypertrichosis may rarely occur as an inherited disorder and occasionally appears later in life, when it may be due to certain illnesses. In such cases detailed medical investigations are necessary to pinpoint the cause, particularly if this is a sudden growth. Anorexia and extreme weight loss through dieting or exercise are often accompanied by profuse growth of fine downy hair on the face and elsewhere.

A curious legend relates to St Wilgefortis, whose father was a king in Portugal in the Middle Ages. He had arranged her marriage to the king of Sicily, but she had become devoutly religious and had decided to remain a virgin. She is said to have prayed and fasted with the result that she developed an excess growth of hair on her face, which her suitor found so unattractive that he withdrew his offer of marriage. Wilgefortis became an early Christian martyr when her father had her crucified as punishment. A statue of this unfortunate woman can be found in Westminster Abbey. She was usually depicted with a beard and a moustache, so in a way can be regarded as the patron saint of hirsute women. If there is any factual basis to this story, the unfortunate girl probably suffered from hypertrichosis as a result of her anorexia.

Some cases of hypertrichosis are due to medication. For example, corticosteroid drugs prescribed for serious or life-threatening illnesses can induce hypertrichosis, but only after very long-term treatment and in high doses. Minoxidil, a drug used to treat high blood pressure, is known to cause hypertrichosis, and this property has been exploited as an external application to promote hair growth in male-type balding (chapter 4). Some drugs used in epilepsy may also cause excess hair growth. Other medications have similar actions to the male (androgen) hormones and produce hirsutism, for example the anabolic steroids used by some athletes.

Hair growth at puberty

During childhood the skin is covered in fine, downy, lightly pigmented hair called **vellus** hair except on the scalp, eyebrows and lashes, where coarse hair called **terminal** hair grows. The pubic and armpit coarse (terminal) hair growth appearing around puberty is known as **secondary sexual hair** since it relates to the appearance of adult levels of sex hormones.

After puberty males develop secondary sexual hair in more extensive areas than females. This is because they are genetically primed this way and because they produce much more androgen than females. What is not generally realised is that females have the *potential* to develop secondary sexual hair in the same pattern as males do—the difference is in the amount and coarseness of the hair. There are large individual and ethnic variations in female secondary sexual hair growth, brunettes tending to have more than blondes. Women of Mediterranean or Semitic origin, with olive skin and brunette colouring, usually have more pronounced body and facial hair than fair or blonde women, although there are exceptions. Asian women usually have very little facial and body hair.

What is normal?

What exactly is a 'normal' amount of body or facial hair in a woman? To a large extent this is determined by the society in which she lives—and to some extent what the women's magazines decide is normal! Many women whose facial and body hair growth is well within the normal range will perceive themselves as falling well short of the current ideal of feminine attractiveness promoted by fashion magazines. Some teenage girls feel self-conscious about fine downy hair on the upper lip, particularly if the hair is dark, whereas this is quite normal during pubertal development. Similarly, coarse hair in the sideburn area is normal in certain racial groups and a majority of brunette women normally develop hair around the nipples and centre of the lower abdomen. Darker and coarser hairs also develop on the forearms and, even more so, on the lower legs in girls around puberty. However the way androgens influence hair growth in these areas is a very variable trait with some women having only fine (vellus) hairs and others having coarse dark leg hairs and coarser than average forearm hairs. 'Mohair stockings' are just as much part of growing up as are fuzzy armpits and pubic hair!

Furthermore, most adult women do not have a neat triangle of pubic hair conveniently capable of being covered by high-cut bathers—extension of the pubic hair into the groin and upper inside thighs is actually normal. Hence there is a distressing contrast between reality and the hairless smooth-skinned models of glossy magazines and cosmetic advertisements.

Excess body and facial hair is only very rarely due to a hormonal problem. It is estimated that only 1–2 per cent of women who consult doctors because of excess hair have a serious hormonal (endocrine gland) disturbance. In the majority, hirsutism is an inherited feature, more common in women with dark hair and eye colouring and hence more likely to be found in certain ethnic groups. The medical term for this is **simple hirsutism**. It only becomes a problem if the woman *perceives* herself as abnormal in relation to those around her. This fact is often sadly exploited by the cosmetic and beauty industry.

In some cases, the doctor will order blood and urine tests to establish whether or not the hair growth is due to an excess of androgen hormone. Such investigations are likely to be needed if the hirsutism is severe, or has appeared suddenly and has worsened rapidly, or if there are accompanying irregularities in the menstrual cycle. These would include severely irregular or completely absent periods. In fact, it is not uncommon for women with simple hirsutism to have slightly irregular periods without this in any way signalling a serious hormonal imbalance. This simply highlights the fact that, as with many aspects of biological functioning, there is a wide spectrum of variability in the menstrual cycle and the cyclic production of hormones. There are also individual and racial variations in the way the target for androgens in our skin, namely the pilo-sebaceous unit, responds to these hormones. This alone explains why no two women have identical amounts of facial and body hair.

It is not uncommon for women with hirsutism to suffer from acne both in the teens and the mature years. This is not surprising since we know that both problems are based on increased sensitivity of the pilo-sebaceous unit to stimulation by androgen hormones.

In rare cases where over-production of androgens is the cause of increased hair growth, a woman may show signs of actual masculinisation (or virilisation), such as deepening of the voice, receding scalp hair line, decreased breast size, increase in muscular development, and enlargement of the clitoris. Such changes certainly signal over-production of androgens and should sound alarm bells. Causes include tumours of the ovaries or adrenal glands and other rare malfunctions of the endocrine system. Fortunately this does not apply to the majority of women who complain of hirsutism.

How is hirsutism treated?

Dealing with the emotional aspects

Some women with hirsutism need initially to deal with the problem at the psychological level. Many simply do not realise that their hair growth falls within the normal range and may feel greatly reassured when this is explained to them. Others have a genuine problem with how they perceive their bodies. They regard what may in reality be a minor problem as a major cosmetic handicap. Body image distortion, similar to that occurring in some forms of anorexia and bulimia, may play a role in some cases.

Practical methods of hair camouflage and removal
These are are dealt with in chapter 4.

Treatment of hirsutism with medication
Anti-androgen drugs work in hirsutism by blocking the androgen receptor so that androgen circulating in the blood and produced in the skin cannot stimulate the hair follicle to grow. The result is decreased hair growth rate plus lighter and finer hair. This change occurs slowly over several months of treatment. In most cases there is a continued need for hair removal by whatever is the preferred method, although with greatly decreased frequency.

The areas where hair is most sensitive to androgen stimulation (chin, neck and upper lip) respond best to treatment with anti-androgen medication. The thighs and pubic area are the least responsive in most cases, and forearm and lower leg hair is usually not reduced much by anti-androgen treatment. There is also an unpredictable variability in the response of individual women to this treatment. Some show excellent improvement within six months of commencing treatment, while others notice only marginal improvement after twelve months. Unfortunately it is not a permanent cure for excess hair since the effect of blocking the androgen gradually falls off once the drug is ceased. After several months the hair growth usually returns to its former level.

Cyproterone acetate and **spironolactone** are the two anti-androgen drugs currently in use in the treatment of acne (chapter 2). They can also be used to treat hirsutism. Both need to be given under strict medical supervision and should not be used in pregnancy. Cyproterone acetate needs to be taken with oestrogen in women who still have menstrual periods. It can be given by itself in women who have had a hysterectomy or who are past the menopause. The oestrogen can be conveniently given as an oral contraceptive and hence cyproterone acetate is an ideal form of treatment for hirsute women who are already on the Pill. Spironolactone does not need to be given with oestrogen and so can be used in women who do not need or want the Pill, or who have some medical reason to avoid oestrogen treatment. Cyproterone acetate can also be incorporated into a hormone replacement regime in post-menopausal women who require treatment for hirsutism.

Six to nine months treatment with anti-androgens is usually needed to achieve maximum suppression of hair growth. Courses of around two years would usually be the minimum period, but some young women may elect to continue for much longer, perhaps at reduced dosage, provided no pregnancy is planned. Anti-androgens are in general well tolerated, although there may be some minor side effects such as sore breasts, mild fatigue and irregular or light periods.

Treatment with anti-androgens is obviously not the complete solution for the problem of unwanted hair, but it can be very useful for women who want to take positive steps to suppress hair growth even if it is only a temporary solution. It can be particularly effective if combined with electrolysis and regular waxing, and if expectations of the results are not too unrealistic.

ORAL CONTRACEPTIVES AND THE SKIN

Pigmentation of the face

Pigmentation of the face, known as **melasma** (or **chloasma**), occurs in some women taking the Pill and is also common in pregnancy. It is thought to be due to oestrogen somehow reacting with ultraviolet rays since it doesn't occur unless there is also sun exposure. It is more likely to be a problem in women whose skin tans easily. Unfortunately it also occurs quite frequently in women who are neither pregnant nor taking oral contraceptives or any other type of oestrogen medication.

Melasma can be reduced gradually with a cream or lotion containing the bleaching agent hydroquinone. It can be combined with isotretinoin to enhance the effect. A disadvantage is that this may cause skin irritation and the application must be gradually increased so that skin tolerance develops. It is also extremely important to avoid sun exposure as much as possible. Even broad spectrum sunscreens do not provide complete protection against the UVA rays which seem to be especially responsible for this type of skin pigmentation. Mild peels induced by glycolic acid can also help lighten melasma (see chapter 9).

Antibiotics and oral contraceptives

The contraceptive effect of the birth-control pill may be reduced if antibiotics are taken at the same time. This is thought to be caused by the effect of the antibiotic on the absorption of oestrogen from the bowel. Some women experience breakthrough bleeding as a result. This is a sign that the oestrogen blood level has fallen and consequently there is an associated risk of ovulation occurring. Although many antibiotics have been implicated, tetracyclines, which are so frequently used in treatment of acne, are among the most common. This effect tends to wear off after the first month of combined treatment and is less pronounced with lower doses of antibiotic. There are a few other medications which may affect oral contraceptives—so it is important for the prescribing doctor to know what other drugs you are taking.

Thrush occurs more frequently in women on oral contraceptives (see chapter 5).

Acne in most cases improves when the oral contraceptive is taken because of the beneficial effect of oestrogen. Oestrogen acts on oil glands, reducing oil production, and it also acts by a more complex influence on androgens in the bloodstream. Some women seem to suffer the reverse effect, with worsening of acne. This may be due to the progestogen in the Pill which, in most oral contraceptives, is levonorgestrel. This progestogen has some androgen-like qualities, but the way the progestogen exerts its influence at the sebaceous gland is a highly individual effect varying from one woman to another. In women with this problem, two alternatives are available. One is to switch to the oral contraceptive Diane 35 ED which contains cyproterone acetate as the progestogen instead of levonorgestrel. The anti-androgen effect of cyproterone acetate helps prevent acne. The other alternative is to switch to a pill containing a progestogen which has no androgen-like effect.

Hair loss in association with the Pill is discussed in chapter 4.

Spiders (dilated capillaries) also occur more frequently in young women taking the oral contraceptive as well as during pregnancy. (See page 67.) They also frequently occur in girls who are not taking hormones, especially around or just before puberty.

THE SKIN AND THE MENSTRUAL CYCLE

Some women notice increased oiliness of the hair and skin just before each period. Acne may worsen at this time for many women. We do not know precisely why this increased oil gland activity happens at this time of the cycle. The female progestogen hormone produced from the ovary in the second half of each monthly cycle may have an effect similar to androgens in stimulating oil glands. In addition, stress may influence the part of the brain known as the **hypothalamus**. The hypothalamus produces chemicals which in turn stimulate the adrenal gland causing it to make more androgens. It is also possible that increased water retention around the oil ducts during this part of the cycle may aggravate pore blockage. Women who are not already using an oral contraceptive and who suffer from pre-menstrual acne flare ups will usually improve when an oral contraceptive is used. This is mainly because of the beneficial effects of the oestrogen in the Pill. (See page 51). An even better approach is to take the Pill that contains the anti-androgen cyproterone acetate (Diane 35 ED), which has a beneficial affect on acne throughout the whole monthly cycle.

Some pre-menstrual women experience flushing episodes rather similar to menopausal hot flushes. Pre-existing skin disease such as psoriasis and eczema may worsen just before the period.

BABY ON BOARD: PREGNANCY AND YOUR SKIN

Most women go through pregnancy without serious skin problems. Having a child means that life is never the same again. Your skin also changes, but in more subtle ways. Some of these changes may be permanent.

Skin pigmentation

Deepening of skin pigmentation is common around the nipples and on the vulva, and also occurs in a line from the navel to the pubic area. This pigmentation is more pronounced in brunettes and olive-skinned women and only partially fades after childbirth.

Many pregnant women also notice an increase in the number of moles on their skin and a darkening of moles already present. Some of these 'moles' are not true moles but are warty growths called seborrhoeic keratoses (see chapter 9). They often occur between and in the creases of the skin below the breasts. Of course, any significant change in pigmentation or size of a mole should be reported to your doctor.

Melasma (or chloasma), also known as the 'mask of pregnancy', is blotchy, symmetrical pigmentation on the face similar to that occurring in some young women, sometimes in relation to oral contraceptive medication (see page 63). Melasma may spontaneously improve or disappear completely after delivery, and it is certainly made worse by unprotected sun exposure.

All these pigmentation changes in skin are said to be due to the increased oestrogen levels in the bloodstream during pregnancy, but the cause is by no means certain. It is possible that other pigment-stimulating hormones (perhaps originating in the pituitary gland, which is an endocrine gland in the brain) may increase in pregnant women. In addition the placenta produces hormones—not yet fully identified—which probably play a role in these and other changes in the body during pregnancy.

Other skin problems in pregnancy

Many pregnant women develop a 'healthy glow', with general improvement in skin and hair especially during mid and late pregnancy. Acne often improves, and some women notice that scalp hair grows more quickly. The complex hormonal changes of pregnancy, particularly the high oestrogen levels, may result in decreased androgen stimulation of sebaceous glands, causing a decreased tendency to acne. Unfortunately, in some women, acne may inexplicably worsen—more commonly in the early stages of pregnancy. In these women it has been shown that, in spite of the high blood levels of oestrogen, sebum production may actually increase. This increase in sebaceous gland activity may continue during breast feeding. Again it is suggested that hormones produced by the pituitary gland may be responsible.

Oestrogen also affects small blood vessels in the skin. **Spider naevi** occur in around 70 per cent of pregnant women. They consist of radiating blood vessels extending from an enlarged central blood vessel and are most pronounced on the face, neck and upper chest. Most disappear spontaneously after pregnancy but some may persist. If cosmetically embarrassing they can be treated with fine needle diathermy (see chapter 9) or laser treatment (chapter 10). Some women develop spiders in the same areas in subsequent pregnancies.

Reddening of the skin of the palms is also common during pregnancy. Sometimes the whole palm is affected, sometimes just the borders of the palm. As part of this general stimulation of the growth of small blood vessels in the skin, some pregnant women develop small harmless blood vessel 'tumours' called **pyogenic granulomas**. Whilst they are not dangerous, they occasionally bleed profusely and need surgical removal, usually by curettage. **Swollen red gums** in pregnancy are thought to be related to the general increase in blood vessels in the mucous membrane. It is important to attend to oral hygiene to prevent gingivitis (inflammation of the gums).

Spider veins (also known as 'venous flares') are unpleasant purple surface networks of small veins on the leg. Many women attribute these to pregnancy, but they are just as common in women who have never been pregnant and also occur in men. Fortunately they can be removed with sclerotherapy (see chapter 9). On the other hand, **varicose veins** may worsen or appear for the first time during pregnancy, as may haemorrhoids, which are similar. They may also affect the vulva. Aching tired legs may result from problem varicose veins. Deep vein thrombosis is a potential serious complication. Whilst the exact cause of varicose veins is not known it is thought to be an inherited defect resulting in weakness in the valves or the walls of the veins—this being exaggerated by the hormonal changes of pregnancy and the pressure of the enlarging womb. Whilst varicose veins occur in men, they are about three times more common in women.

Itchy skin without a visible rash (known as *pruritus gravidarum*) occurs in around 1 in 200 pregnancies, mostly in the later stages, and often occurs mainly over the abdomen. It is thought to be due to changes in bile production in the liver caused by the high levels of hormones in the bloodstream during pregnancy. Fortunately it usually disappears rapidly after birth, but it can be intensely irritating. Antihistamine drugs (those cleared as safe in pregnancy) and cooling anti-itch applications and baths may be needed.

An itchy skin rash in the last stages of pregnancy, usually with the first baby, occurs in around 1 in 300 pregnancies. Dermatologists call it the **polymorphic eruption of pregnancy**. The itching and rash usually first appear on the lower abdomen overlying stretch marks, but then spread to the arms and thighs. Its cause is still a mystery but it certainly has no sinister implications and in no way affects the health of the mother or baby. It disappears quite rapidly after birth, but when severe may need to be treated with steroid creams, anti-itch applications, and carefully selected antihistamines.

Women who suffer from eczema or psoriasis may notice dramatic improvement during pregnancy, but unfortunately this is unpredictable and some actually worsen. Likewise pregnancy may have an adverse effect on autoimmune diseases like lupus erythematosus.

Cracked nipples during pregnancy and breastfeeding can be a particular problem for women who suffer from atopic eczema, but also sometimes occurs in the early stages of lactation in women who have had no previous skin problems. In most cases simple emollients (moisturisers) or low strength steroid ointments cure this problem. So-called 'natural' remedies are also popular, possibly because women tend to shy away from anything which smacks of 'artificial' medication at this time.

Stretch marks, known medically as striae, are not, contrary to popular folklore, simply due to the stretching of the skin by the enlarging womb. They are thought to be due to a hormone produced by the adrenal glands, since they are also common in people with overactivity of that gland (Cushing's Syndrome). They are also very common in adolescence in body areas where body fat increases at this time, such as the thighs, buttocks and breasts. They are also common in adolescent boys in areas such as the thighs and buttocks. Stretch marks are due to changes in the connective tissue of the skin, and appear in parts where increase in size occurs relatively rapidly. In pregnancy they appear on the breasts, buttocks and thighs as well as on the abdomen. There is *no* satisfactory treatment. Fortunately they often fade in time but can be cosmetically unsightly, particularly in the early stages when reddish/purple in colour. Isotretinoin cream has recently been reported to improve striae but has obvious drawbacks since it cannot be used in pregnant or breastfeeding women because of the risk of absorption through the skin and consequent damage to the foetus or baby. It is a complete waste of time to massage creams, oils and vitamin preparations or any of the other many suggested treatments alleged to prevent pregnancy stretch marks.

Skin tags (small cauliflower-like growths) and **seborrhoeic keratoses** may increase in numbers and size in pregnancy, particularly between and under the breasts and in the armpits. Many are small and disappear spontaneously after pregnancy. Those which do not can be removed simply, usually with liquid nitrogen therapy or surgical removal followed by diathermy. (See chapter 9.)

The hair in pregnancy is discussed in chapter 4.

THE MENOPAUSE AND YOUR SKIN

The menopause or last menstrual period occurs at any time between the ages of 45 and 55. The years leading up to this event and immediately following it—the **peri-menopause** or 'climacteric'—are associated with some changes in the skin, some subtle, others dramatic. Approximately 1 per cent of women experience menopause prematurely, under the age of 40, and some women are precipitated into a premature menopause if the ovaries are surgically removed, such as for tumours or endometriosis. When the cyclic release of eggs from the ovaries (ovulation) ceases there is also a decrease and eventual cessation of their hormone-producing function, with the result that oestrogen levels decline. This does not happen overnight—blood levels of oestrogen may fluctuate quite dramatically over many years before finally falling to a permanently low level. Women past the menopause continue to produce *some* oestrogen but it comes from chemical conversion of hormones produced in the adrenal glands. These conversions take place in the skin and body fat.

Along with the decline in oestrogen production at the menopause, androgens normally formed in the ovary also decline. The adrenal glands, on the other hand, continue to produce androgens. The continued formation of these androgens, combined with the lack of oestrogen, results in the androgen hormones exerting a greater influence in tissues sensitive to them. It is therefore not surprising that *some* of the unwelcome skin changes which occur after the menopause in women are partly due to excess androgen stimulation. These problems include hirsutism, peri-menopausal acne, and androgenetic hair loss (see chapter 4).

No two women are likely to experience the same skin changes at the menopause because genetic factors are very important and changes in hormone levels themselves are likely to vary enormously from one woman to another.

Hot flushes

Once the monthly cycles of hormone production from the ovaries cease, the complex signalling system from the ovary to the pituitary gland in the brain also ceases. This leads to increased levels of hormones produced in the pituitary called **gonadotrophins**. Before menopause, these gonadotrophins are critically important in controlling the ovary's production of hormones and ovulation. It is thought that one of these gonadotrophins, **follicular stimulating hormone** or FSH, may partly be responsible for hot flushes. These are the best known and most discussed symptom of the menopause, occurring in at least 50 per cent of women.

Hot flushes vary in severity, from a mild sensation of warmth lasting seconds to minutes to distressing episodes lasting several minutes or longer. They may be accompanied by blotchy flushing of the face, neck and chest skin, sensations of intense heat, profuse sweating, and even palpitations, nausea and anxiety. Hot flushes and night sweats may precede the menopause by some years and continue well afterwards. Although this phenonemon is much more complex than simple oestrogen deficiency, oestrogen replacement therapy usually reduces the symptoms, although not always completely. Many women will experience some relief from hot flushes when taking placebo tablets—containing no actual hormones—suggesting that other factors are involved. This may also explain why natural and alternative therapies benefit some women. However, well controlled studies do tend to show that oestrogen therapy is beneficial in most cases.

Does menopause affect the quality of your skin?

At the same time as oestrogen levels are declining at the menopause, changes related to *chronological ageing* as well as the first signs of chronic sun damage (*photoageing*) are emerging. It is difficult to be certain exactly how oestrogen lack fits into the scenario. Oestrogen deficiency after the menopause is thought to contribute to *some* of the ageing of our skin, particularly skin dryness, thinning of the epidermis (the top layer of our skin), and breakdown of collagen in the dermis leading to the loss of skin elasticity. There is some evidence that oestrogen treatment in women leads to thickening of the dermis over time, but the effects on epidermis are not clear. It is likely that HRT (hormone replacement therapy) has some beneficial effects on skin by increasing the thickness of collagen and perhaps decreasing its breakdown. On the other hand *no amount of extra oestrogen will reverse the degeneration of skin due to photoageing and it will not remove wrinkles.*

Many menopausal women notice a dramatic increase in overall dryness of the skin, particularly in the areas of skin which may have formerly been oily, such as the T-zone of the face. The lower legs may become dry and flaking, photoageing also being an important factor in this area. On the body, dryness may contribute to sensations of *itchiness*. This is usually relieved by water dispersable bath oils and suitable moisturisers. If unchecked, eczema patches may develop; common sites for this are on the back, between the shoulder-blades and on the lower legs.

Hard, dry callused heel skin with a tendency to form cracks may become apparent in middle-aged women. This is more related to mechanical factors than oestrogen lack, being more often seen in overweight women and those who habitually go bare-footed.

There is *absolutely no evidence* that hormones such as oestrogen and progesterone in cosmetic creams exert any beneficial affect on the skin or relieve dryness any more effectively than moisturisers not containing hormones. Furthermore, as hormones in creams are actually absorbed through the skin into the blood stream (which is precisely why oestrogen patches work), the net effect is like taking a small dose of oestrogen orally.

ACNE IN MENOPAUSAL WOMEN

After the menopause, sebaceous gland function decreases but some women experience a sudden breakout of acne at this time. There are three possible reasons for this. As the skin becomes noticeably drier, many women succumb to the pressures of the cosmetic industry to purchase often expensive moisturisers and in some cases over-use of these oily creams causes 'acne cosmetica'. This is partly due to the blockage of sebaceous glands and partly due to a chemical reaction induced by ingredients in cosmetics that encourage blackhead formation. Another reason is that, although androgen production from the ovary declines along with oestrogen production, androgens to some extent assume a more dominant role in some skin areas. Very few of these women have abnormal amounts of androgen in the bloodstream but it seems that, at least in some menopausal women, the sensitivity of the pilo-sebaceous unit to androgen stimulation is somehow heightened. Hirsutism is one result and acne is the other. A third reason is that in some women the progesterone hormone in their HRT combination may have a slight androgen-like effect. This can be likened to the way in which a *minority* of young women on oral contraceptives experience a worsening of acne (see page 64). It should be emphasised that the way in which individual women metabolise hormones varies greatly so this is not an important effect in all women.

Menopausal and peri-menopausal acne may improve simply by switching to oil-free moisturisers and cosmetics. Remnants of cleansing cream left on the skin can also block sebaceous glands and encourage blackhead formation. Washing with a good mild soap will solve this problem. Antibiotics may be needed in severe cases of acne. Another option is anti-androgen treatment. This can be incorporated into an HRT regime by substituting **cyproterone acetate** for the progestogen. **Spironolactone** can be used in women not on HRT. In peri-menopausal women still menstruating and still needing contraception, a solution is to use the oral contraceptive containing cyproterone acetate (Diane 35 ED) with the option of adding extra cyproterone acetate if the acne remains severe. A considerable amount of fine tuning may be needed in individual cases and this requires careful medical supervision. A minority of women with cystic acne at the menopause may need isotretinoin oral therapy.

Hirsutism at the menopause

Facial hair tends to increase at the menopause, probably because of the more dominant role assumed by androgen in sensitive skin areas. Women with no previous problems may suddenly sprout coarse hair from the chin and coarser hair on the upper lip. Eyebrows may thicken with the appearance of longer darker hairs. As in younger women, social conditioning will largely determine how well a woman is able to deal at the emotional level with this unwanted hair problem. Anti-androgen drugs can be used, with or without HRT, and the usual methods of camouflage and removal can be employed (see chapter 4). Medications prescribed for various medical problems occasionally cause excess facial hair as an inconvenient side effect—for example some drugs used to treat epilepsy. Oral steroids in prolonged courses over many months or years can also cause facial hair but this is of a more diffuse and fine type (hypertrichosis rather than true hirsutism).

Rosacea

Some 'acne' around the middle years of life is not acne at all but an acne-like condition called **rosacea**. Rosacea is common in both sexes in the late forties and fifties and also involves inflammation of sebaceous glands, but there are none of the blackheads or whiteheads which are so characteristic of true acne. It may start with episodes of flushing of the face in the 'butterfly area' of the nose and cheeks which eventually develops into a permanent redness. On this background inflamed pimple-like spots develop, and at the same time the persisting flush aggravates any tendency to 'broken' capillaries on the cheeks. The flush is exaggerated by alcohol, heat, caffeine and anxiety. Germaine Greer in *The Change* (Hamish Hamilton, London, 1991) suggests that the menopause is a good time to abandon old addictions, and there is certainly some evidence that women with rosacea benefit from reduced alcohol and caffeine intake. Since sunlight also exacerbates rosacea, sun protection is important. The condition is more common in fair skin of Celtic type, which is also more prone to sun damage.

Whilst the cause of rosacea is not known, a small organism which normally resides in the sebaceous gland-rich T-zone of the face, known as *Demodex folliculorum*, has been implicated. Metronidazole, which eradicates this organism and can be applied in the form of a gel, benefits most cases. More severe cases respond to tetracycline antibiotics but these may need to be given for a prolonged course of several months or more.

Peri-oral dermatitis is a condition *related* to rosacea which mainly affects young women but sometimes emerges for the first time in the years leading up to the menopause. This rash consists of tiny grouped pimples occurring mainly around the mouth and on the chin. The cause is not known but the same condition may develop when strong cortisone applications are used on the face. Fluoridated toothpastes, cosmetics and hormonal factors (for example oral contraceptives and pregnancy) have also been implicated. A course of tetracyclines usually cures the condition within around six weeks, although relapses may occur.

Poikiloderma of Civatte is the name dermatologists use for a very characteristic combination of pigmentation and fine dilated capillary networks that occurs predominantly on the sides of the neck in peri-menopausal and older women. There is usually a pale area under the chin where the skin is protected from the sun. Dermatologists so far have been unable fully to explain this annoying skin mottling although sun exposure plays some role. There is no satisfactory treatment.

HRT and the skin

Are there any skin problems caused by HRT? Some women develop skin irritation from HRT patches which is alleviated by changing their position frequently. Sometimes a true allergic contact dermatitis develops, making the HRT patch an impossible option. Some women develop melasma (see page 63) when on HRT and in combination with sun exposure. Sun protection is important to minimise this, and if necessary medically prescribed depigmenting lotions and creams can be used.

THE ELDERLY WOMAN'S SKIN

In old age the sex hormones which exerted a significant influence on certain areas of our skin in the decades from puberty to menopause are no longer active. Blemishes which may proliferate on the skin at this time are by no means confined to females.

The earliest signs of photoageing (see chapter 9) start to appear in the fifties or even earlier. Skin cancers are more likely to appear in later life. Solar lentigines (large irregular flat freckles) appear on the face and hands. As the collagen in skin degenerates, bruising occurs easily on the exposed areas of the hands and forearms, resulting in large purplish bruises which seem to 'come from nowhere' after very minor knocks and scrapes.

Seborrhoeic keratoses and skin tags start appearing in increasing numbers (chapter 9). Many women put on weight at this time, and this seems to encourage growth of skin tags around the armpits and sometimes in the groin. They are also common under and between the breasts and on the neck. A frequent complaint is that they rub on clothing or catch on necklaces etc.

A recurring nuisance, particularly in overweight women, is a red itchy rash under the breasts, in the groin and other skin folds, called **intertrigo**. (See chapter 5.) Moisture and sweating in the warm skin folds encourage the yeast *candida*, resulting in the complication of thrush. Treatment is targeted at alleviating the sweating by using drying powders and wearing clothing which allows the skin to breathe, and is also aimed at reducing inflammation and clearing up the thrush.

Hair tends to decrease in most areas except the face, and some women develop coarser eyebrow hairs. Many women discover to their extreme exasperation that whilst they no longer need to worry about hair removal on the legs or armpits they now need to don their bifocals to pluck stray hairs from their chin.

Apocrine sweat glands become less active in old age, so sweat odour usually becomes less of a problem. Nails thicken and become ridged. Itchy skin associated with dryness and exaggerated by cold weather and low humidity can be a problem for some older women. Water-dispersable bath oils are helpful. It is also helpful to use less soap and aim to use mild unperfumed soap or to apply emollients immediately after bathing and towelling dry. Moisturisers containing 10 per cent urea, glycerine and olive oil are all effective in aged, dry skin.

In later life **cherry angiomas**, which are also called 'Campbell de Morgan spots' start appearing in increased numbers. These are bright cherry red raised or flat spots consisting of collections of tiny, dilated blood vessels. They vary in size from pin point to a few millimetres in diameter, and occur mainly on the trunk from middle age on. They tend to disappear in very old age. The tendency to dilated blood vessels (**telangiectases**) on the cheeks and nose becomes more exaggerated in the elderly as the skin becomes thinner and less elastic. Elderly women may develop dilated veins, called **venous lakes,** on the lips, causing bluish swellings which can look quite alarming but are not dangerous. Likewise, the venous networks or so-called **starburst vessels** on the legs are exaggerated as the ageing skin becomes thinner.

There are methods available to remove or at least significantly diminish many of the unwelcome blemishes that proliferate on the skin as a result of ageing and photoageing. These are discussed in chapter 9. Potentially dangerous spots should be treated on medical grounds. As for the innocent or benign blemishes which are of only cosmetic nuisance, then this is up to the individual. Many middle-aged and ageing women are not concerned about minor blemishes. They believe, quite rightly, that they have earned their wrinkles and skin spots and are entitled to keep them! In *The Change* Germaine Greer writes of 'secret marks of age, the witch marks' which could be seen 'if we were to be hauled off and stripped naked at our own witch trial'. But she urges us to have the last word against the ageists and 'assume the witch's right and cackle in our turn'.

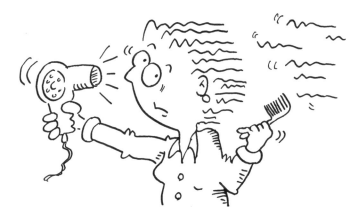

CHAPTER FOUR

CROWNING GLORY

A guide to hair problems

JILL CARGNELLO

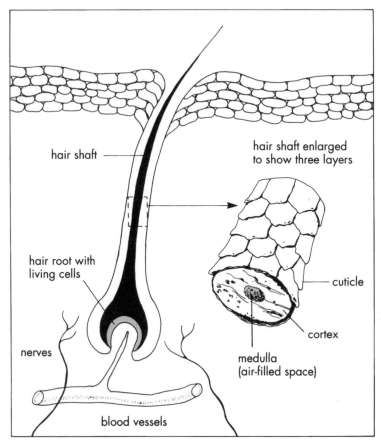

hair shaft

hair shaft enlarged
to show three layers

hair root with
living cells

nerves

cuticle

cortex

medulla
(air-filled space)

blood vessels

Hair follicle in active growth phase (anogen)

Over thousands of years of evolution human body hair has
become increasingly irrelevant as a barrier against the cold
and elements. Despite its relative sparsity it has profound
social and psychological importance. The ancient Egyptians
wrote about hair restoration lotions and twentieth century
men continue to search for the elusive baldness cure.

Broadly speaking there are only two hair disorders: *too
much*, and *too little*!

In order to understand the common problems which can
affect our hair and scalp you need some basic knowledge of
the structure of our hair and how it grows.

HAIR STRUCTURE

Each hair shaft is elliptical or circular in cross-section and is composed of three concentric layers. The core, known as the **medulla**, is little more than an air-filled space running down the centre of each hair. Surrounding this is the **cortex**, which makes up most of the bulk of the hair and is composed of a tough fibrous protein called **keratin**. The cortex is in turn surrounded by an outer layer known as the **cuticle**. The cuticle consists of six to eight layers of flattened cells which overlap each other in much the same way as roof shingles overlap. The cuticle is extremely hard and forms a protective covering around the hair shaft. See diagram.

The fine downy hair which covers most of the body is known as **vellus** hair. Unlike the coarse thicker hairs (known as **terminal** hairs) that sprout from areas such as the scalp, eyebrows and pubic area, vellus hair is short, virtually colourless and has no medulla. If you look on the inside of your forearms you will see typical fine vellus hair.

The quality of hair is determined by minor variations in the hair shaft. For instance, straight hair is perfectly circular in cross-section whereas wavy or curly hair is more slender and elliptical. Negroid hair is flattened and ribbon-like, giving its characteristic tightly coiled quality. The condition of the cuticle determines how light is reflected from the hair. When the cuticle is badly weathered and individual cells stick out or are lost, or if the cuticle is covered by grease and dust, the hair appears dull and lifeless. If the cells are overlapping and lying flat against each other like a neatly tiled roof, light will be reflected evenly from this smooth surface and the hair will appear glossy and smooth.

HAIR GROWTH

Our hair does not grow continuously. It has cycles of growth followed by rest periods. During the growth phase (**anagen**) the hair shaft is being formed within the depths of the hair follicle. It is firmly attached to the base of the follicle and cannot be pulled out without causing pain. It has a dark or pigmented root and its own tiny blood vessels which provide the hair root with all its nutritional requirements. The hair root is the only part of the hair which is composed of living cells. The actual hair shaft is not alive, so terms such as 'feeding the hair' and ' nourishing the hair' are nonsensical.

The growth rate of hair varies little between the sexes and among individuals, averageing 1 cm per month. The growth period lasts between 3 to 6 years and this will determine the maximum length of the hair. If you have ever wondered why some women can grow hair down to their thighs whilst you have trouble getting it to grow much beyond collar length it is because your growth cycle lasts about 2 years rather than 7.

In rare cases the inability to achieve long hair is due to excessive weathering of the hair resulting in breakage of the hair shaft. This may be due to some abnormality of the hair structure, something a person is born with. It can also be due to extreme over-processing of the hair, such as too frequent perming, bleaching and over-drying with electric hair dryers.

When the anagen period is over the hair stops growing and the follicle enters its resting period (**telogen**). The hair root loses its attachment to the base of the hair follicle and sits much closer to the skin surface. These resting or telogen hairs can be easily and painlessly removed from the scalp by simple brushing and shampooing and are recognisable by their white (non-pigmented) hair root. People who are losing their hair often become very distressed when they notice the white hair bulb at the end of hairs that are shed from the scalp, mistakenly believing that the hair is falling out by the root. Telogen hairs have in fact stopped growing, and they are no longer attached to the living cells at the base of the hair follicle. They cannot re-anchor themselves and start growing again. This means that treating the hair especially gently by hardly ever brushing it or by washing it very infrequently will not help. Sooner or later, these shed hairs will work their way out of the scalp. However the hair follicle is still intact and will grow another hair shaft when the next growth phase begins.

Our hair growth, unlike that of many other mammals, is not synchronised. We shed hair continuously rather than having seasonal moults. Under normal circumstances 50 to 100 hairs are shed daily and should be thought of as replaceable loss. Some people notice little hair loss on a day-to-day basis although most would be aware of increased hair loss on shampooing or vigorous brushing. During shampooing the scalp is rubbed in such a way that telogen hairs are easily dislodged. Other people may notice periods of increased hair shedding for weeks or months at a time sometimes causing enough concern to prompt a visit to a dermatologist. Sometimes this is due to a greater number of hair follicles than usual stopping their growth phase and entering the telogen phase simultaneously (see page 92).

ITCHY SCALP, DANDRUFF AND PSORIASIS

An itchy scalp is often the first sign of dandruff, seborrhoeic dermatitis or psoriasis. In all three dermatological disorders, the individual skin cells on the scalp grow and divide more rapidly than usual. This results in increased shedding of flattened dead cells, called squames, that get caught on the hair shaft or fall onto clothing. To the naked eye, the squames appear as tiny white flakes which stand out most on dark hair or dark clothing. The appearance of these white flakes should not be interpreted as evidence of scalp dryness or of a poor quality shampoo.

Dandruff, the mildest of the three conditions, can usually be controlled with a shampoo containing zinc pirithione or selenium sulfide. Fortunately, such anti-dandruff shampoos are freely available and widely marketed.

Seborrhoeic dermatitis is more extensive and examination of the scalp may reveal pink or light tan slightly scaly patches varying in size from a few millimetres to several centimetres. These patches cannot usually be felt with the fingertips, which helps to differentiate this condition from psoriasis. Recent research has shown that a yeast known as *Pityrosporum ovale* may play a role in causing this annoying problem.

Fortunately, this yeast can usually be eradicated by zinc pirithione or selenium sulfide in concentrations usually found in anti-dandruff shampoos. In resistant cases, your dermatologist may need to prescribe a special cream or shampoo to alleviate the problem.

Psoriasis is usually more severe and characterised by thick crusted plaques which can be readily felt with the fingertips. The plaques are common behind the ears and over the back of the scalp just above the nape of the neck. The plaques themselves are bright pink and have a thick crust of silvery scales. Treatment of psoriasis is considerably more complicated than that for dandruff or seborrhoeic dermatitis and is also influenced by the presence or absence of psoriasis elsewhere on the body. In most instances, the dermatologist will prescribe cream to be massaged into the scalp, as well as specialised shampoos. Creams and lotions containing tar are highly effective in the management of psoriasis but unfortunately tend to stain and smell unpleasant. Cortisone creams and lotions are much more pleasant to use but unfortunately are only suitable for mild cases of psoriasis. Furthermore, with continued use these products gradually become less effective. Recent studies overseas have demonstrated the effectiveness of a new vitamin D cream in the management of scalp psoriasis.

TOO MUCH HAIR

From the medical viewpoint, there are two different types of abnormal increased hair growth: *hirsutism* and *hypertrichosis*.

Hirsutism is medical jargon for increased growth of terminal (coarse, usually dark) hair in skin areas targeted by the 'male' sex hormones called **androgens**. Such areas include the upper lip, chin, chest, pubic area and thighs. Hair growth in these sites is first noticed at puberty and becomes more prominent with age. The vast majority of women with excessive hair in these areas are perfectly normal in the hormone department. In other words they don't have too many male hormones. The problem is simply that their hair follicles are overly sensitive to androgen hormones, the result being darker and coarser hair than usual. On the other hand, if a woman has increased hair growth and in addition has symptoms like irregular periods, deepening of the voice, acne or other signs of masculinisation her doctor will usually need to check the androgen hormone levels. Hirsutism is covered in more detail in chapter 3. Because hirsutism results from androgen stimulation, medication to counteract these hormones can be used to treat it.

Hypertrichosis is the medical name for increased growth of fine vellus hairs in areas such as the forehead and forearms where androgen hormones don't have much influence. Hypertrichosis occasionally occurs due to medication, in particular corticosteroids and Cyclosporin A, or as a manifestation of internal illness. If the hair growth is rapid in onset or vigorous your doctor will need to carry out some tests to pinpoint the cause. Treatment with anti-androgens will not benefit hypertrichosis as it is not due to androgen stimulation.

How to deal with excess hair

If you have unwanted hair and it bothers you enough to want its removal there are both medical (prescribed medications) and physical options available. Medical therapy means using drugs called anti-androgens. Two types are currently available, **spironolactone** and **cyproterone acetate**. There is a delay of 4 to 6 months before improvement is likely and on stopping the medication hair growth gradually reverts to the pretreatment level. Medical therapy does not stop hair growth altogether but it will slow it down and promote the growth of fine vellus hair rather than coarse terminal hairs.

Most women prefer the convenience of and instantaneous results achieved with physical methods of hair removal, such as shaving, plucking, waxing, depilatory creams and electrolysis. There are two types of hair removal, *depilation* and *epilation*.

Depilation is the removal of hair at the level of the skin surface, as occurs with shaving and depilatory creams. The hair shaft is cut at its widest point so the regrowth may feel bristly or coarse. This has given rise to the myth that shaving actually increases hair growth and makes it coarser.

There is no reason to fear that once you have shaved you will be ever after committed to repeating it regularly to deal with an ever coarsening growth. In practical terms, shaving is quick, painless and effective and should not cause ingrown hairs or skin irritation if a good quality razor (electric or blade) is used.

Depilatory creams are composed of chemicals (thioglycolates or sulfides) which bind to the hair shaft and attack keratin protein, weakening it to the point of breakage. As with shaving, the hair is removed at the skin level. Hair keratin is similar to skin keratin, so these creams are extremely irritating, especially if used too frequently.

Bleaching, though not a means of hair removal, is an excellent means of rendering hair growth less apparent, particularly when there is a problem with ingrown hairs or unsightly regrowth. A number of commercial preparations are available for home use.

Epilation is the removal of the hair shaft and its root from the follicle. It may be permanent, as with electrolysis, or temporary, as with waxing and plucking. Removal of the hair root delays hair regrowth by two or more weeks. In contrast to shaving, after waxing and tweezing the new hair emerges with a tapered soft tip, giving the impression of a finer regrowth. Unfortunately the soft hair tip is more likely to curl and pierce the sides of the follicle, giving rise to ingrown hairs.

Electrolysis and thermolysis use low voltage electric current to destroy the living cells at the base of the hair follicle that produce the hair shaft. Although in theory an attractive means of hair removal, results are entirely dependent on the skill of the operator. At best 15 to 25 per cent of treated hairs will regrow. Most operators can remove between 25 to 100 hairs per sitting. This means a woman with moderately coarse beard growth may require years of treatment at three to four week intervals before achieving a satisfactory result. Treatments should be well spaced to allow adequate healing between sessions. Too frequent treatment results in inflamed skin, a tendency to ingrown hairs, acne-like spots, and the risk of pitted scars. Some women with olive toned complexions may develop brown stains in the skin which may be as disfiguring as the original hair problem! Infection is a potential hazard, especially if epilation needles are not adequately sterilised. Responsible therapists should use single-use sterile disposible needles for electrolysis. In summary electrolysis is a reliable method of permanent hair removal but the procedure is tedious, painful and expensive and carries a risk of scarring and infection. So do your research before deciding on your therapist.

Several magazines carry an advertisement for permanent hair removal using a pair of electronic tweezers. The American Food and Drug Administration have found them to be no more effective than conventional tweezers!

Too LITTLE HAIR

Alopecia is the technical term for hair loss. The word itself does not tell us anything about the cause or likelihood of recovery. There are dozens of causes of hair loss recognised by dermatologists; they are all called alopecia. Many people mistakenly believe that the term refers only to a special type of hair loss called *alopecia areata* (see page 89). Fortunately the majority of cases of alopecia are temporary or treatable.

Dermatologists divide alopecia in two main categories. In one type the hair loss is associated with the formation of scar tissue in the skin of the scalp. This is called **scarring alopecia**. It results from various skin diseases, most of which are quite rare, where the degree of damage to the hair follicle is so great that scar tissue forms. This means that the hair follicles are destroyed and the alopecia will be permanent. The hair loss is often patchy and irregular. There may be a red scaly rash, or the scalp in the bald patches may look quite normal, but be firm to the touch. The skin also often has a peculiar shiny and smooth look and when examined closely there are no follicle openings. Usually in these cases the dermatologist needs to carry out complex investigations including a scalp biopsy (the removal of tissue for examination) to find out exactly what is causing the problem. The information gained from these tests is then used to determine the most effective treatment.

Non-scarring alopecia

In **non-scarring alopecia** there is no actual destruction of follicles or scar tissue formation. This means that the follicles are still present, although they may be diseased, altered in some way, or their growth arrested. The alopecia in the non-scarring conditions shows up as an increased shedding of hair leading to gradual loss of hair density and fullness. The hair loss may be all over the scalp, in other words *diffuse*, or it may be in discrete patches or localised mainly over the crown. Recognising various patterns gives the dermatologist clues as to what type it is and what is causing it. The scalp skin can look pretty normal and the openings of the hair follicles can be seen as tiny pores even in the areas which are quite bald.

There are dozens of causes of non-scarring alopecia. Some are associated with general medical problems including infections, auto-immune diseases like lupus erythematosus, thyroid disease, and severe kidney disease. In many of these cases the hair loss is just a minor symptom in relation to the other problem.

A large number of medications may cause non-scarring hair loss as a side effect in a small percentage of people. The best known example are the drugs used in chemotherapy for cancer. In these cases the hair loss may begin within days of starting treatment and can be quite dramatic, sometimes leading to complete baldness. Once the drug or drugs are stopped the hair folicles will recover and the hair will regrow. With many other drugs the hair loss is not noticed for several weeks or months after the medication is started. This often makes it quite difficult for the dermatologist to pinpoint the problem accurately, particularly when a patient is taking several different types of prescribed medications!

Some nutritional difficiences can also cause non-scarring hair loss. Severe protein lack due to malnutrition is one— fortunately rare in our society. Zinc deficiency has also been associated with hair loss and can occur in some rare illnesses in which zinc in food is not absorbed properly from the intestinal tract.

One of the more common nutritional deficiences is iron deficiency. Some women become iron deficient because of multiple pregnancies (and inadequate iron supplementation) or because of heavy periods, or by being completely vegetarian and thus missing out on iron-rich food. Our hair seems to need iron to grow properly and if our iron stores are low the hair may start to thin out a little. If there are other hair loss problems going on at the same time, for example androgenetic alopecia (discussed on page 90) these may be exaggerated by the iron deficiency. This can be easily rectified by taking iron supplements but it must be supervised—a person can take too much!

Alopecia areata (AA)

Alopecia areata is a non-scarring type of hair loss. It is total hair loss in discrete areas. Research now suggests that AA is an autoimmune phenomenon caused by one's own disease-fighting white blood cells (lymphocytes). Rather than complete destruction of hair follicles, the 'attack' results in switching off follicular growth. This means that even though the hair may be lost from most of the scalp there is still potential for complete recovery. Unfortunately, despite much research doctors are still trying to determine what actually triggers this abnormal immune response. Stress may trigger attacks in some people, but hair loss itself is extremely stressful so it is often difficult be sure whether the hair loss preceded the stress or occurred after. Furthermore AA can occur in well, happy children from supportive homes and in well balanced, apparently stress-free adults.

The bald scalp is usually pale and normal in appearance, with no crusting or any skin infection. Occasionally an itching or creeping sensation may be noticed prior to the hair loss but in most people the condition comes on without warning. The bald area may be first noticed by a hairdresser or family member. When alopecia areata remains confined to one discrete area the likelihood of total hair regrowth is good. In most cases regrowth will occur within six months. However, despite full recovery there is a fifty per cent chance of another patch of alopecia areata appearing, often years down the track.

If there are multiple bald patches or if the balding is progressing rapidly then treatment is warranted. In such cases there is a greater risk of developing total scalp and or body hair loss (known as **alopecia totalis** and **alopecia universalis**), with a poorer outcome and less likelihood of full recovery. Sometimes people with AA get nail changes, for example, tiny pits in the nail plate or separation of the nail plate from the nail bed (onycholysis).

The type of treatment used in AA will depend on the age of the person involved, the extent of the hair loss, and the rate at which hair loss is progressing. The dermatologist may use cortisone in tablet, cream, lotion or injectable form to dampen down the abnormal immune response. She may also choose a non-cortisone based lotion or cream deliberately designed to cause irritation of the scalp. The purpose of this form of treatment is to divert the abnormal immune response from the hair follicle to the skin surface, thus stimulating hair growth again. Some people find the resulting irritation and rash too unpleasant and are not likely to put up with it for long if it does not produce results. Other people with severe AA might consider the inconvenience a reasonable trade-off for the hope of some regrowth, particularly when other treatment methods have failed. We certainly don't have all the answers yet for this puzzling and sometimes distressing condition.

Androgenetic alopecia (MPA)

Androgenetic (or male-pattern) alopecia is a hereditary form of hair loss that occurs in both males and females and is also a non-scarring type. It is caused by androgens (male hormones). Paradoxically the hormones which stimulate hair growth on the body cause progressive hair thinning on the scalp. The hair on the temples, crown and sometimes the sides of the scalp gradually becomes finer, downy and sparse. MPA in women, as opposed to that in men, does not result in complete balding. This is due to the protective role of oestrogen (female hormone). Hair loss and thinning may first become apparent at puberty in males but usually not until the twenties in most women. It progresses at a variable rate. In addition, women do notice some general thinning of the hair with age quite apart from MPA. This is just a normal part of the natural ageing process.

In a small number of women, the onset of MPA may be associated with menstrual irregularity, severe acne, increased body hair, or enlargement of the clitoris, all signs of a potential excessive production of androgen hormones. This combination of symptoms usually requires further investigation by a medical practitioner.

As it is an inherited or genetic disorder there is no cure for MPA despite the multitude of 'hair restoring' lotions and potions on the market. **Minoxidil** lotion (Regaine) is the only preparation currently available which has been proven to stimulate hair growth. Twice daily application of a 2 per cent solution of minoxidil can bring about cosmetically acceptable (i.e. noticeable) hair regrowth in 30 per cent of users. It usually takes 4 to 6 months to see a response. The most accurate assessment can really only be made after a whole year of use. Women with mild hair thinning tend to benefit most from minoxidil.

Spironolactone and cyproterone acetate are medications used in the treatment of MPA in women. These compounds block receptors on the hair follicle that are normally stimulated by androgen hormones and in doing so prevent the latter from having an influence on follicular activity and hair growth. A beneficial effect is noticed in up to 60 per cent of women. Neither is suitable for use in men because of their anti male hormone effect. Most males, even if worried about hair thinning, would not consider loss of libido and masculinity an acceptable trade off!

Telogen effluvium

Telogen effluvium is increased shedding of resting (telogen) hairs. It is caused by various triggers capable of shunting actively growing hair follicles into telogen with subsequent shedding of hairs. There may be a delay of 1 to 4 months between the trigger or stimulus and the increased hair fall. As a result the initial triggering event may go unrecognised. High fever, major illness, childbirth, anaesthetics and weight loss may provoke telogen effluvium. Typically the hair loss reaches a peak 6 months after the initiating event. Recovery occurs spontaneously and completely within a few months, although sometimes there are complicating factors which delay recovery. One of the commonest of these is iron deficiency.

Hair loss following childbirth varies a lot. It is usually quite mild and most women are so busy caring for the new baby that they don't even notice it. In other women it might be so severe that it prompts a visit to the doctor. It usually comes on 2 to 3 months after the birth and usually recovers completely within 6 to 12 months. Occasionally if a woman has several pregnancies in quick succession it may never completely recover. Strangely enough it may not follow every pregnancy in the one woman and it has nothing to do with the sex of the baby. It is believed that the sudden fall in oestrogen levels at the end of the pregnancy causes large numbers of hair follicles to enter the telogen phase of the growth cycle simultaneously.

The Pill and your hair

There are two ways in which the Pill can cause hair loss but it only occurs in a small percentage of women. One type of hair loss is thought to be due to the synthetic progestogen which may have an androgen-like effect, particularly in those women who have a genetic susceptibility to develop androgenetic alopecia. This problem was more common in the 1960s when the doses of the hormones in the Pill were high by today's standards. It does not happen in all women because no two women react to hormones in the same way.

The other type of hair loss occurs when the Pill is ceased and is rather like the hair shedding which follows childbirth (telogen effluvium, described above). It is usually not a severe hair loss and is not permanent. Anyone noticing this can be assured that the hair will return completely to normal within 5 or 6 months.

HAIR COSMETICS AND SALON TREATMENTS

Hair cosmetics encompass shampoos, conditioners and hair colouring agents.

Shampoo and conditioners

A good **shampoo** should be capable of removing the build-up of oil, dead skin cells and atmospheric pollutants that bind to the hair shaft, and it should rinse cleanly from the hair and scalp. Soap will cleanse the hair, but in hard water areas may lead to a build-up of insoluble soap salts or scum which impart a dull appearance to the hair. Shampoos utilise synthetic detergents which are less likely to have this problem. Acidic shampoos (low pH, 4.5 to 6.0) cause less swelling of the hair shaft and roughening of the cuticle and do not disturb the acid mantle of the skin. Consequently these are preferred if the hair is already damaged or if you have a tendency to develop eczema.

Shampoo manufacturers include a variety of additives including herbal extracts, natural oils and conditioning agents to make their product more appealing. These add little to the actual performance of the shampoo and in the case of the 'conditioning' shampoos may even reduce its effectiveness.

Conditioners act as detanglers and make the hair softer and more manageable, and reduce static electricity. When applied after shampooing they leave a film on the hair which smoothes down the hair cuticle. They may even fill in deficiencies in the cuticle and temporarily seal split ends together. Proteins and silicone are particularly good at transiently adhering to the hair shaft and are incorporated into conditioners for this purpose. Unfortunately no product can permanently repair split ends. The only 'cure' for damaged hair is to cut off the damaged portion.

In summary the function of a shampoo is to strip the hair of undesirable residues whilst conditioners leave a thin invisible film on the hair, two opposing functions which are difficult to combine in the one product. Combined shampoo and conditioners inevitably lead to accumulation of detergents and are best reserved for occasional use. A separate shampoo and conditioner will do a better job of both cleaning and conditioning.

Hair colouring products

Almost 50 per cent of women and a growing percentage of males are dissatisfied with their natural hair colour. If you are considering a change of hair colour it is worthwhile having some knowledge of how this may be achieved.

There are five basic types of hair colour: gradual, temporary, semipermanent, permanent, and bleaches.

Gradual hair colourants are most frequently promoted as a way of restoring colour to grey or white hair. These dyes are composed of metallic salts that are rubbed onto the hair daily until shades of brown and black gradually appear. These preparations are not messy and are easy to use but have several disadvantages. They smell unpleasant, and because the metal salts are deposited on the outside of the hair cuticle they make the hair look dull and lifeless. In addition their presence precludes the use of permanent waves or colouring because the chemicals used in these other processes cannot penetrate the layer of metal salts coating the hair shaft. Finally these dyes cannot be removed from the hair shaft without causing hair damage and should be left to grow out.

Temporary hair colouring can be achieved with the use of synthetic compounds that are deposited on the outside of the hair shaft. These products are available as rinses, mousses, gels and sprays, and can be used to tone down brassy tones in bleached hair or to give a new but temporary party look—particularly when shades of green, blue and purple are used!

These dyes wash out with one shampoo. If the user is unfortunate enough to be caught in the rain the dye will run and stain both skin and clothing.

Semi-permanent hair dyes are the most popular form of hair dye and are used both at home and in hair-dressing salons. These dyes penetrate the cuticle (the outer layer of the hair shaft) to the hair cortex and will withstand 6 to 10 shampoos. They are most commonly used as a means of brightening or subduing natural or bleached hair colour. They do not interfere with permanent waves or other hair processing. They are readily obtainable from chemists and supermarkets and are simple to use. These dyes rarely cause allergic contact dermatitis and can usually be tolerated by people who are allergic to permanent hair dyes.

Vegetable dyes are another form of semi-permanent hair colour, and are derived from plants such as Roman or German chamomile, logwood, walnut, and the North African shrub *Lawsonia alba*. Henna, which is used to give the hair rich red or auburn tones, is derived from the dried leaves of the latter. These dyes stain the cuticle and do not penetrate the hair shaft. They will not radically alter hair colour but can be used to accentuate hair colour and blend in grey hair. Like synthetic semipermanent dyes they have the advantage of washing out after a few shampoos and do not interfere with other hair processing.

Permanent hair colouring is so named because the dyes actually penetrate the hair shaft and form large colour molecules that become trapped within the hair cortex. They cannot be removed by shampooing. Re-dyeing is necessary every 4 to 6 weeks to deal with the regrowth at the scalp. Permanent (or oxidative) hair colouring generates a complex chemical reaction within the hair shaft between the dye and a developer (also called an 'oxidising' agent). This results in the formation of a large colour molecule. The developer is usually hydrogen peroxide, which has the additional effect of bleaching the natural hair colour as the new colour is being developed.

Permanent hair dyes are also known as **para** dyes or **amino** dyes because they contain paraphenylenediamine

(PPD) or closely related chemicals. PPD can cause allergic contact dermatitis in up to 10 per cent of users. Furthermore, allergy may develop even after numerous trouble-free applications of these dyes. It is consequently recommended that the dye be applied to a small test site on the nape of the neck or forearm prior to applying these colourants. If the test site becomes itchy or red the para dyes should not be used.

Unfortunately the bleaching reaction which takes place within the hair shaft damages the keratin. As a result repetitive applications of permanent dyes can cause damage and breakage of the hair shaft. Dyeing should not be carried out more frequently than every 3 to 4 weeks and the dye should only be applied to the regrowth.

Bleaching

Bleaching is a means of lightening hair colour. The hair pigment melanin is chemically changed by an oxidising agent, usually hydrogen peroxide. The hydrogen peroxide is mixed with an alkaline ammonium solution immediately prior to application to speed up the reaction. Both the oxidising agent and alkaline ammonium are damaging to hair keratin, rendering the hair dry, porous and more prone to tangling. The increased porosity of the hair allows bleached hair to absorb more water, resulting in longer drying times and increased susceptibility to humidity changes. The bleached hair will also take up semipermanent and permanent dyes and waving preparations more easily. This means weaker solutions should be used on bleached hair.

Hair permanent waving solutions

There are three types of naturally occurring wave patterns in human hair: straight, wavy and kinked. The straight hair shaft is circular and is most typified by Asian hair. Wavy hair is oval and is the most common Caucasian hair form. Kinked hair is tightly curled and breaks easily, as in African hair, which is elongated or ribbon-like in cross-section.

These genetically inherited patterns can be altered by breaking the chemical bonds in the hair in what is known as a softening process. The hair can then be reshaped around rollers in the desired style and then another chemical applied to reform the broken chemical bonds so that the hair will retain its altered shape. In practice it is impossible to reform all of the broken hair bonds so the treated hair will always be weaker and more brittle. Furthermore, as one can imagine, permanent waving is by nature extremely damaging to the hair shaft.

Cold waving solutions have almost entirely replaced the older hot waving techniques. The latter used heat in the reshaping stage, and had a greater propensity to cause excessive hair shaft damage.

Hair straighteners

The principal of hair straightening is much the same as permanent waving. Hot combing or cold chemical solutions can be used to achieve the desired straightening of the hair shaft. Hot combing involves the application of vaseline or oil to the hair, which works as a heat transferring agent, then the use of a heat press or hot comb to straighten the hair. Temperatures of up to 97°C are used in the process. Small wonder that this often results in severe weathering and breakage of the hair!

Cold chemical straightening involves the same processes and reactions as permanent waving, using cold chemicals rather than heat.

Hair extensions

Hair extensions are a popular way of adding length to the hair. The extension is composed of human or synthetic hair depending on budget and the look one is trying to achieve. The extension is attached to the pre-existing hair by a combination of braiding and wax. Extensions are secure enough to withstand gentle shampooing, hair styling and swimming, and may be expected to last for between three and four months if properly cared for. As extensions are applied to the ends of the hair shaft they add length rather than volume, so are not a solution for men and women with androgenic alopecia.

Dreadlocks

Dreadlocks are strands of matted hair that usually form naturally in individuals with wavy or kinked hair. Instead of being shed, telogen hairs become caught up in the wavy locks where they then add to the obstacles preventing other telogen hairs being shed cleanly from the scalp. These hairs then become caught up along with sebum, dead skin cells and atmospheric pollutants to form thick cords of matted hair. The development of dreadlocks is encouraged by infrequent washing, minimal or no combing, and twisting of the developing 'locks'.

TRICHOLOGISTS, HAIR CLINICS AND HOPE

It is hardly suprising, given the important role our crowning glory plays in our self image, that the most common initial reaction to hair loss or hair disease is sheer panic, followed by a visit to the chemist, hairdresser or neighbour for some type of remedy. If the problem persists a visit to a trichologist, commercial hair clinic or doctor usually ensues. Unfortunately many individuals end up in the hands of unscrupulous dealers who see hair disorders purely as a means of generating income, and may find themselves several months down the track considerably poorer with no end in sight to the original hair problem!

When seeking help for a hair problem, ask the advice of someone who knows something of hair physiology and general health. Your hairdresser may be able to offer advice or treatment for brittle or damaged hair, but if the problem is one of excessive hair loss or scalp disease your local doctor should be the first point of reference. Your doctor can assess your general health and the role medication may be playing, and he or she is unlikely to sell you a little tonic whipped up in the back room which is conspicuously lacking in label and ingredient list! If your doctor is uncertain as to the cause of the hair problem, ask for a referral to a dermatologist who has spent years studying diseases of the skin and hair.

Some people prefer to seek the advice of a trichologist, which literally means 'one who studies hair'. Your dermatologist, doctor, hairdresser or motor mechanic may have legitimate reason to assume this title. The title 'trichologist' does not imply the completion of a formal academic qualification and only by asking exactly what qualifications your trichologist has will you determine his or her fitness to deal with your problem.

Under no circumstances sign contracts for courses of treatment based on advice or threats suggesting that unless active therapy is started immediately the problem will be impossible to rectify. The more pressure that is applied to have you commit financially to any form of therapy the more scepticism it should generate. Effective treatment does not need heavy selling!

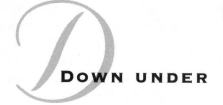

CHAPTER FIVE

DOWN UNDER

Genital skin problems in women

TANJA BOHL

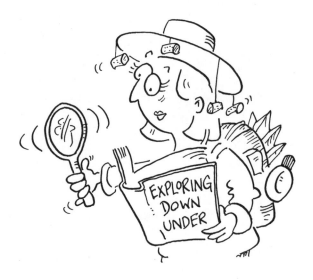

Why a chapter about the female genitals in a book about skin? A gynaecologist I know describes the vulva as 'the frontier where our two specialties meet'.

The **vulva** is the anatomical name for the female external genital area. It is lined on the outside by skin and on the inside by specialised skin and also by mucous membrane. As a result the vulva can be affected by a variety of skin diseases which go beyond what is covered by most books concentrating on the gynaecological aspect of women's health. Common skin diseases like eczema and psoriasis can affect any part of the skin, including the vulva. On the other hand, there are some skin problems to which the vulva is particularly prone, for example lichen sclerosus (page 114). There are some rare diseases which affect *only* genital skin, in both men and women. Diseases which specifically attack mucous membranes can turn up here. Finally, the side effects of some drugs sometimes focus on the genitals.

Doctors researching and treating vulval diseases by no means have all the solutions. There are vulval diseases which continue to pose more questions than provide answers!

The chapter concentrates on the common skin diseases not only because they *are* common but also because, as you come to understand these problems, you will also learn more about this area of your body.

WHAT IS NORMAL?

In women the external genitals are hidden between the thighs, making them impossible to see from above. Because the openings of the bladder (**urethral meatus**), vagina (**introitus**) and bowels (**anus**) are close together, we are taught to clean carefully after going to the toilet by wiping ourselves from the front to the back. This helps create the myth very early in life that this area of our body is not only mysterious and invisible, but dirty.

Women rarely have the opportunity to see the variations which can occur from one individual to another. Therefore we are likely to worry if our genital area looks a bit different from what we might see in text books or in the media.

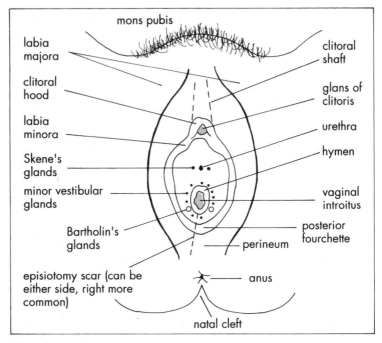

The vulva

Understanding the proper medical names given to the genital area helps us understand what our doctors and other health professionals tell us. It will also help us to explain our problems to our doctors if we know the right names, and avoid potential embarrassment and confusion. In the diagram the main anatomical structures are labelled.

If you wish, you can use this as a guide for examining your own body, although it is not compulsory or necessary in order to understand what follows. Set aside a time and place where you can be guaranteed not to be interrupted. You will need a hand mirror. Sitting on a firm surface with your back supported and your pelvis tilted forwards is probably the most comfortable position. Pull your knees up and put your heels together and then let your knees fall out to the sides as far as is comfortable. You may hold the hand mirror in one hand and use the other to explore your body, or you may choose to prop it up either against your feet or on an extra pillow so that you can see clearly.

Pubic hair is very variable from one woman to another. In general the hairs are thicker, curlier and coarser than those of your scalp, and they can even be a different colour. In women of Mediterranean descent they are usually very thick and very extensive. They can extend onto the inner thigh and around the anus and onto the buttocks. Asian women tend to have much less pubic hair. As women grow older and past menopause the amount of pubic hair, as well as underarm hair, reduces dramatically and can sometimes disappear altogether.

The **labia majora** (literally 'large lips') are the outer lips which touch along their edges when we stand. When they do this they form a covering over the vulva. This creates a warm and moist environment—an important point to remember because it can influence skin problems in this area. These warm, moist conditions explain why some skin diseases, for example psoriasis, look quite different on the vulva as compared with other skin areas. The main bulk of the labia majora is fatty tissue. In older women they tend to shrink and become thinner. The outside of the labia majora looks like normal skin and is covered by pubic hair whereas the inner surface is shiny and hairless.

Inside the labia majora are the inner lips (**labia minora**). Starting from the front near the mons pubis the inner lips form the **clitoral hood**. The little knob which is the visible part of the clitoris is called the **glans clitoris** or head of the clitoris. This is the most sensitive sexual part of our anatomy. Whilst this can be a great source of pleasure in the right circumstances, inflammation around this area can be a great source of discomfort. If you gently feel the tissue above the clitoris you will feel a little ridge of tissue deep inside. The tissue here becomes swollen or engorged with blood when we become sexually aroused.

The labia minora or inner lips vary a lot in size and in colour, and also become engorged when we are sexually aroused. In some women the tiny oil glands there are visible as little yellow dots along the edges of the labia minora. Moving in further, we find the opening of the bladder (**urethral meatus**). On each side of this are glands which help in lubrication called **Skene's glands**.

Below this we find the vaginal opening (**introitus**). The **hymen** which separates the vulval area from the vagina varies enormously from woman to woman. It may be a nice neat complete rim but sometimes it is fragmented, even from birth. Sometimes it may seal off the vagina completely, a problem which is usually picked up when women first start menstruating. Period pain and discomfort will occur monthly but there will be no blood loss and a lump forms at the entrance to the vagina as menstrual blood builds up. After childbirth the hymen may be totally disrupted with very little left. On the outside of the hymen, on either side and just a little bit towards the back of the vulva, are the openings of the **Bartholin's glands**. These are also a source of lubrication. Other lubricating glands occur in a ring around the vaginal entrance—and are called **minor vestibular glands**.

The whole area enclosed by the labia minora from the clitoris in front to the point where the labia minora merge at the back (known as the **fourchette**, which literally means fork) is known as the **vestibule**. The space between the fourchette and the anus is called the **perineum**. This is very variable in length from one woman to another.

In the diagram I have drawn the line along which episiotomies or cuts are most commonly made during childbirth. Episiotomies may distort the anatomy a little, although proper correction at the time of childbirth will usually result in a virtually invisible scar. The cleft between our buttocks (**natal cleft**) is lined by skin similar to that of the rest of our body whereas the skin at the anus is rather like that of the labia minora.

We perspire from ordinary sweat glands in the creases of our upper thighs and around the pubic area. We also have special sweat glands on the vulva which are stimulated by hormones (see chapter 2). This fluid seems to play some role in sexual attraction.

The vagina is a hollow tube lined by specialised skin which contains no mucus glands and also, surprisingly, has no sensory nerves from about 5 cm inside. This means that sensation inside the vagina can be quite different from other parts of the body and largely results from stretching of the wall rather than from stimulation of the actual vaginal lining. At the end of the vagina is the cervix.

FEMALE GENITAL MUTILATION

The normal anatomy is severely distorted by female genital mutilation. In societies which practise female genital mutilation the degree to which the genitals are mutilated varies. In its mildest form it involves removal of the clitoral hood. Sometimes the clitoris is also removed.

In its most severe form the clitoral hood, clitoris and labia minora are all removed and the labia majora pulled together to close the wound. A small hole is left through which urine and menstrual blood escape.

These procedures are usually done without any anaesthetic. Depending on the culture or religion involved, the age of the woman undergoing this mutilation varies. It is often done around the age of puberty. It is also often done in grossly unhygienic conditions.

The risks to the young women involved depend on who performs the procedure, where it is done and the method used, and can include severe pain, bleeding, infection and death.

Sexual enjoyment after anything but the most minor of these procedures is lost or at least severely impaired. In the most severe cases sexual intercourse may not be possible at all without opening of the vulva by cutting. In some societies special knives are provided to husbands for this purpose on their wedding nights. Childbirth can pose a potentially life-threatening situation for both mother and child due to the degree of scarring which can occur.

There are no medical reasons for these procedures.

VAGINAL DISCHARGE

What is normal?

Amount and type of discharge varies greatly from one woman to another. It will be affected to some degree by whether or not she is on the Pill, and also whether or not she has had recent intercourse or sexual arousal. In women who are not on the Pill the discharge tends to be thin and very sparse in the early part of the cycle just after the period. As ovulation approaches the discharge becomes more profuse, and at the time of ovulation it becomes thick and sticky. Recognising these changes is an integral part of using cervical mucus examinations in the Billings method of contraception. As we enter the latter stage of our menstrual cycle the discharge will become more profuse but less sticky.

Some birth control pills tend to even out these changes in vaginal discharge. Even when on the Pill some women notice differences from one time of the cycle to another even though ovulation is not occurring. These changes tend to be more obvious in women who take the sequential oral contraceptive in which the dose of hormone varies from one part of the cycle to the other.

The amount of sex hormones in the blood varies during our menstrual cycle. These cyclic fluctuations in hormone levels determine the cyclic changes in our vulva and can, in turn, influence certain skin problems which occur in this area.

Natural vaginal odour varies from one woman to another and also during our menstrual cycle. Alterations in odour can occur with certain problems, for example a musty or sweet odour is often associated with thrush and a fishy odour may occur with some other infections. Be aware of what is normal for you as it will help you to recognise these problems if they occur.

VULVAL ITCHING

The most common symptom complained of by women in the genital area is *itch*. This can vary from an occasional irritation to an insistent and constant itch which prevents sleep and hampers day-to-day activities. It may make work, shopping and social outings a nightmare. All the affected woman has on her mind is the availability of the nearest toilet to which she can rush for a good scratch! Some women scratch to the point of producing small ulcers or sores and will often say that a bit of pain in this area, or even a lot of pain, is better than the constant itch and irritation.

Naturally, an inflamed vulva, with broken skin areas, will smart and sting when urine is passed. Women should be frank about giving details of all these symptoms to their doctor, otherwise the doctor might simply focus on the burning feeling on passing urine and diagnose a bladder infection.

THE THRUSH STORY

Our vulvas and vaginas normally contain a lot of bacteria and a small amount of the yeast *candida*. These organisms comprise what is known as the 'normal flora'. In other words having them there is OK, it is the normal state of affairs.

Potentially problem-causing bacteria can be easily introduced into the vagina from the nearby anus. Our vagina fortunately has its own defences to guard against this, as it is normally bathed in an acidic liquid containing bacteria called *Lactobacilli*. By keeping the environment on the acidic side, these 'friendly' bacteria discourage 'unfriendly' bacteria as well as keeping candida in check.

Many of us will be aware that **thrush**, due to overgrowth of candida in the vagina, can be triggered by taking some antibiotics. This is because the normal friendly or protective bacteria in the vagina are killed off by the antibiotic, resulting in a breakdown of the defence system. This allows the candida yeast to flourish.

Iron deficiency also predisposes to thrush. Women who have had successive pregnancies without taking enough iron supplements, or who have very heavy periods, or who are exclusively vegetarian, may be more vulnerable to iron deficiency. Women who are diabetic are also more prone to thrush—even those with well controlled diabetes. Women whose immune system is compromised by immunosuppressive drugs or diseases such as AIDS are also at risk.

Thrush is a common problem and its main symptom is itch. In severe cases it can cause a thick white cheesy discharge described as Ricotta cheese-like. The main parts affected are the vagina and the vaginal entrance, which becomes red and raw, and feels rough, hot and burning. Intercourse is uncomfortable or impossible. A doctor can usually diagnose severe thrush of this type from the symptoms and by making an examination, but in addition a swab is sometimes needed.

Sometimes the thrush infection only affects the vulva and not the vagina. In these cases there may not be much discharge at all. The vulva may go through cycles of becoming red, swollen, itchy and painful, commonly with splitting of the skin at the fourchette, particularly after intercourse. These symptoms may be worse in the week before the period.

Fortunately there are some very effective treatments for thrush. Nystatin or various medications of the type known as **imidazoles** usually relieve symptoms when applied as cream or pessaries inserted into the vagina. Nystatin can also be taken as an oral tablet. When taken orally it reduces the amount of candida in the bowel but because it does not actually get absorbed into our system it is not so useful on its own. The idea is that if candida is reduced in the bowel it is less likely to travel from the anus to the vulva and cause problems.

Some women with very stubborn thrush may need to continue treatment for several weeks, even months. Newer oral drugs such as ketoconazole and fluconazole are actually absorbed into our systems and can be used in severe or very chronic cases. Progestogen hormone (Depo-Provera) injections are also useful in difficult cases.

If a woman with thrush has intercourse, her partner may experience some mild itch or irritation for a few days. It is unusual for thrush to persist in a man if he is otherwise well. It is very unlikely that thrush would be passed from partner to partner and back again. The partners of women who get thrush are usually not treated, but if they have some irritation they may be prescribed an anti-thrush cream. Candida is also present in our mouths and oral sex can be another way of spreading the yeast.

Anti-candidal diets are of doubtful benefit. They are designed to reduce the amount of yeast we eat in food, yet food yeasts are not at all the same species as our vaginal yeast. Some women certainly say that they *feel* better on yeast-free diets, but this could be due to other factors quite apart from the avoidance of yeast. For example many women lose weight on these diets, which could well contribute to a feeling of well-being, and there could also be a strong placebo, or psychological, benefit.

ECZEMA OF THE VULVA

Itching and burning on the vulva can be caused by eczema (dermatitis), of which there are two main types, **irritant** and **allergic** (see chapter 7).

Eczema can cause dramatic changes in the skin of the vulva. These vary from tiny blisters, open sores, swelling and redness in the acute forms, through to a dull redness with scaling, thickened skin and cracks in the chronic forms. Because the vulva has such a rich blood supply it is particularly prone to swelling.

A lot of chemical substances and physical factors can act as irritants on the vulva. The most common offenders are listed in Table 1. Once a dermatitis of this type has developed the damaged vulval skin becomes more sensitive to all sorts of other chemicals and physical irritants. This can lead to a vicious cycle. Often substances applied in an attempt to relieve symptoms act as irritants in turn and make things worse.

Some women go to surprising, even alarming, lengths in their efforts to relieve vulval itch. For example, bathing the area in high concentrations of antiseptic, outside manufacturers' guidelines, can produce a profound irritant dermatitis. Not only does this make symptoms worse, it can totally mask the actual problem and make diagnosis impossible until the irritation settles.

In allergic contact dermatitis, there may be a considerable delay between the time when a woman starts using the offending product or substance, and the actual development

Table 1   Irritants in vulval dermatitis

Chemical	Physical
retained sweat	sanitary napkins/tampons
urine	tight clothing
soaps/detergents	toilet paper
deodorant sprays	over zealous cleansing
wart treatments	shaving/plucking hair
disinfectants	intercourse
douches	condoms
lubricants	
spermicides	
perfumes	
saliva	
semen	

Table 2   Subtances which may cause allergic contact dermatitis on the vulva

Local anaesthetics
Local antibiotics
Topical antihistamines
Nickel, e.g. in jewellery
Preservatives in creams
Lanolin
Deodorants
Contraceptives: condoms, spermicides
Clothing: nylon stockings (dyes)
Perfumes
Nail polish
Fabric softeners
Semen

of the skin problem. Again the picture can become extremely complicated because once the vulva is affected by dermatitis it is then more prone to further irritation and allergy. Sorting out what is what can be a daunting problem for the dermatologist. Table 2 lists substances that are frequently the culprits in allergic contact dermatitis of the vulva. Allergies of this sort are confirmed by patch testing, which is discussed in chapter 7.

Atopic eczema is dealt with in chapter 1. People with this skin problem often have a dry sensitive skin which is more prone to irritation, and their vulval skin is no exception.

A special form of eczema called **seborrhoeic eczema** can affect the genital skin. It is a greasy, scaly rash, occurring mainly in the creases of the groin and on the labia majora. Whilst the cause is unknown, dermatologists suspect that perspiration and friction in the body folds play a large role.

How is eczema of the vulva treated?

The basic principle is to avoid substances which can irritate this delicate area—avoid soaps, deodorants and antiseptics. Simple salt bathing is very effective for relief of itching (page 121). It is preferable to pat dry gently with a soft towel—no rubbing. A hair dryer on the cool setting also helps dry the area thoroughly.

If you or your doctor discover that you are allergic to some substance, never use it again. Your dermatologist or gynaecologist will also probably need to prescribe a mild cortisone cream or ointment to clear the rash. Make sure you know exactly how and when to apply it, and how long you should continue to use it.

PSORIASIS OF THE VULVA

Psoriasis is discussed in chapter 1. When it affects the genital area it mostly occurs on the hairy skin of the labia majora and pubic area. Psoriasis can look different in the genital area. When we stand, the entire vulva tends to be enclosed by our thighs and becomes a warm and moist environment. This can alter the psoriasis so that the scaliness goes and we are left with just red patches. You and your doctor can get clues as to whether it is psoriasis by knowing if you have psoriasis elsewhere on your body or whether there is a history of psoriasis in your family.

Spots of psoriasis in the genital area can become cracked. This may be the result of scratching, or from friction from walking or rubbing against clothing. Intercourse also causes irritation. Psoriasis also tends to spring up or 'seed' into areas of skin which are damaged. If you injure the genital skin or develop a rash from some other cause, psoriasis may seed into the area. When the first problem resolves the other may come to the fore!

A note of caution! A new symptom or sudden increase in itch which does not go away with your usual treatment could be a sign of a totally new problem. Superficial skin cancer, for example, can attack the vulva and its only symptom may be itching in the early stages. A dermatologist or gynaecologist recognising such a change in the appearance of the rash will usually need to carry out a biopsy (see page 120). Remember if something does not get better or if something changes—ask why!

INTERTRIGO

Intertrigo is the medical term for inflamed skin in any body fold. It can, for example, affect the skin under the breasts or under the arms.

There are some factors which make certain women more likely to develop intertrigo, for example being overweight and thus having bigger body folds. This encourages perspiration to collect and causes friction as one skin surface moves against another. In the genital skin in particular this can occur simply by the act of walking. Tight, non-absorbent or synthetic clothing also helps increase the heat and friction. Loose cotton underwear is preferred for women with vulval problems of all sorts.

A small degree of urinary incontinence is not uncommon as women age. The muscle around the urethra (the tube that goes from the bladder to the vulva) is influenced by oestrogen. Lack of oestrogen after the menopause contributes to this problem. Childbirth and heavy work can also contribute to prolapse of the bladder leading to incontinence of urine. The urine then irritates the skin and keeps the area moist and hence more prone to friction and infection. Mild incontinence or leakage of bowel movements (faeces) may also occur. Because of the proximity of the anus to the vulva the soiling may spread onto the vulva, taking certain bacteria with it. In this way infection with bacteria and candida can complicate an otherwise simple sweat rash, or indeed any of the other skin diseases discussed so far.

LICHEN SCLEROSUS (ET ATROPHICUS)

This is one of the most common diseases dermatologists and gynaecologists treat at the specialised vulval diseases clinics. 'Sclerosus' means deep thickening within the skin. 'Et atrophicus' means that there can also be thinning of the skin, or atrophy. The name tells us a lot about what the condition looks like. Because it is such a long name it is abbreviated to **LS**.

One of the earliest changes is that the oil glands on the labia minora start to fade and disappear and the labia minora seem to become attached to the inside surface of the labia majora. With time they may disappear completely. Whitening of the skin is very common and some areas become thick and firm. Very prominent blood vessels, called **telangiectasia,** can be present on the surface and sometimes these bleed. Blisters and ulcers can also occur.

In time the vulva may come to look abnormal—like a white sheet with an opening, much smaller than normal, in which you can see the entrances to the bladder and vagina. At this point other problems like splitting and tearing with intercourse and perhaps even problems urinating are likely. The main symptom of LS is *itch*. We do not know what exactly causes this itch. Some women with only very minor LS have quite intense itch, and others with more advanced changes have hardly any symptoms at all.

It was once thought that LS was mainly a problem of older women, but it is now realised that it can strike women in their 20s and 30s and even children. The youngest case reported so far has been a six-week-old girl. This raises another important issue. It is clearly important that doctors examining the vulva in young girls in whom the question of potential sexual abuse has been raised are aware of this condition as it is one that could be confused with child sexual abuse.

The cause of LS is not known but we do know that it tends to run in families. We also know that about 15–20 per cent of women with the condition will get it on other parts of their skin. We also know that occasionally men get it on the foreskin and glans of the penis. The most plausible theory is that the body's immune system produces auto-antibodies against part of the skin and that these abnormal antibodies trigger the disease.

How is lichen sclerosus treated?

Strong cortisone creams used in short bursts under medical supervision not only take away the symptoms but can also improve the abnormal skin. The earlier the disease is treated the greater the improvement. Cortisone creams are safe provided your doctor supervises treatment and provided they are used for the right reason. You should be examined regularly by your doctor so that an experienced eye can be kept out for any early changes signalling the need to reduce the amount or change the type of cortisone cream.

Skin cancer is known to develop very occasionally on the vulvas of women with LS. This may be signalled by a persistent area of pain, itch or ulceration. This is another important reason why women with LS should have regular reviews by their treating doctor as, when detected early, this type of skin cancer can be cured.

MOLES AND OTHER BROWN MARKS

After childbirth or any minor surgery in the area, some women develop flat, pale brown marks on the vulva. These occur around the surgical scar or, after childbirth, in a ring around the vestibule. This discolouration is due to stretching and injury to the tissues that results in pigment cells releasing their pigment and producing a type of tattoo. Uncommonly the number of pigment producing cells in the vulva is abnormally increased, resulting in unusual, irregular flat moles in this area.

In addition ordinary moles of the type that can occur anywhere on our skin (see chapter 8) can occur on the vulva. Women who have a lot of moles on other parts of their body, particularly large, irregular, 'dysplastic' or 'atypical moles', or women who come from families who have a lot of irregular moles and possibly melanoma, should remember that they can also get moles on their genital area. Whilst melanoma is extremely uncommon on the vulva, if you have other factors in your family history or a past history that may increase your risk of developing a melanoma, do not be surprised if your doctor asks you questions about any pigmented areas on the vulva. Have a look yourself if you are not comfortable about being examined. If you find any brown spots or moles, please have them checked!

SEXUALLY TRANSMISSIBLE DISEASES

Sexually transmissible disease (STD) is a term used for diseases caused by germs that most commonly spread by sexual activity. They include conditions like herpes and wart virus infection, as well as gonorrhoea, chlamydia, syphilis and pubic lice (crabs). Condoms provide the best protection from these diseases. A full discussion of these conditions is beyond the scope of this book; however herpes and wart virus infection are particularly important issues because of the concern and emotional distress that they can generate.

Wart virus infection

Warts are caused by a virus called the human papilloma virus (HPV). There are over 80 types or strains, and new ones are being identified all the time. Each different strain prefers to grow in certain areas of skin and is rarely found in others.

HPV has been the subject of a lot of confusion and misinformation. When the HPV infects the skin it may cause a wart to grow, but it can be present in the skin without causing warts. Almost all of us will have HPV on some part of our body, but many of us will never have had a wart.

HPV passes from person to person and place to place by skin-to-skin contact. In the genital area most HPV is associated with sexual contact. It was once thought that warts around the anus in children always meant sexual abuse had occurred, but this has been shown not to be so. (See chapter 1.)

When we come into contact with a new type of HPV we may grow warts two to three months later, but most commonly nothing will happen. A wart may never grow, or one may grow later if there is a reason for our body's immune system to be depressed, for example sickness, stress, or if the skin is broken.

A wart in the genital area is usually found as a lump that is not sore but may occasionally be a bit itchy. Even though a wart is mainly a cosmetic nuisance, genital warts are usually associated with sexual activity so screening for other sexually transmitted diseases is recommended.

Warts may be treated in lots of ways, including freezing, paints, and burning (diathermy). Treatment helps to remove the wart but does not remove all the HPV from the skin. This is why warts may regrow after the initial treatment.

Certain types of HPV, usually the ones that do not grow warts, have been associated with cancer of the neck of the womb (cervix). This is why we should all have regular Pap smears.

A lot of the controversy over HPV in recent times has been about 'silent' infection of the vulva. A woman may have no obvious warts or any history of having warts in the past, and the same may be true for her past and present sexual partners, but when skin from the vulva is removed by biopsy and examined by a histopathologist there may be changes suggesting that HPV is present. In some of these cases no actual HPV is detectable, but most women who have been sexually active have some HPV that can be detected on their vulvas. Most virgins do not have any HPV present. Some confusion exists about what these changes mean, and their relevance must be evaluated in each patient individually.

Herpes

The herpes simplex virus (HSV) belongs to the family of herpes viruses that cause chickenpox, shingles and glandular fever. It is a delicate virus that needs direct skin-to-skin contact to spread. There are two types of HSV—type I and type II. About 95 per cent of 'cold sores' on the face are due to HSV I, and 70 per cent of 'cold sores' on the genitals are due to HSV II. Some overlap occurs.

Most of us are exposed to the HSV type I within the first five years of our lives, usually without any sign of infection as our bodies develop an immune response to the virus and prevent it from producing any illnesses. Sometimes, the first contact with the virus can produce multiple ulcers in the mouth and a general unwell feeling similar to that of a severe cold. This is known as a 'primary attack'. The virus can be spread to other parts of the body by touching a virus-infected area. While this is not common it usually occurs on the fingers, but it can also occur on the buttocks and sometimes the genital area.

The virus always remains within the infected areas and can be reactivated in the future, for example with stress, before your periods, and sometimes by sunlight. These sores are what we know as 'cold sores'. They often start as an area of itch or tingling or burning and then a group of small blisters develop. The blisters then dry and heal over. The whole process usually lasts 7 to 10 days.

A similar situation occurs with herpes virus infection in the genital area. Most genital herpes is acquired sexually, often with no symptoms or with symptoms so mild that the person doesn't realise that they have herpes. A small number of people may develop multiple ulcers on the genital area or feel unwell—a primary attack. Most genital herpes is a reactivation of herpes acquired at some time in the past. This may just be a recurring irritated area or a split in the skin, or look like a typical cold sore. Recurrences occur in the same spot and this is an important clue to the diagnosis.

Some women can have genital herpes and shed the virus, yet feel perfectly well. The only time they realise they carry the infection is if their partner develops a primary attack.

Testing for herpes is done by taking a sample from an ulcer or split for culture. This is best done within the first 24 hours of its occurring. Blood testing is usually not helpful.

Women who have genital herpes can have children normally, but it is important to be tested to see if the virus is active when the baby is ready to be delivered. If it is, a Caesarian section may be done so the baby does not contact the infected area. If the virus is not active a normal delivery is possible.

There are many local treatments that can help soothe the attacks of herpes. Adopting a healthy lifestyle will also help. Although we cannot cure herpes, effective medicines are available to help suppress the virus in people who have multiple recurrences of genital herpes. With time, in otherwise healthy individuals, the attacks naturally become milder and less frequent.

As with genital warts, if you develop genital herpes it is recommended that you have a full screen for other sexually transmissible diseases.

Most major cities in Australia now have specialised clinics to deal with sexually transmitted diseases on a confidential basis. Specially trained medical and paramedical professionals are available to help patients with these problems. These centres are also a very good source of valuable information if you are concerned about any aspect of your sexual health.

VULVAL PAIN

Over the last 10 to 20 years increasing numbers of women have been presenting for treatment at the various specialised vulval diseases clinics complaining of vulval pain, and yet when the doctor examines the patient there is usually very little to see. The pain can be constant, burning and intense, making intercourse difficult or impossible. This is a very frustrating problem for patients and a challenging problem for doctors!

Certain patterns of pain are emerging which are enabling researchers to separate women into groups which share common experiences. This is helping provide clues as to the cause of their problems and ways to treat them.

Some types of vulval pain are limited to the vestibular glands (page 104) which may be inflamed. This is called **vulvar vestibulitis**. Many researchers believe that in this condition skin nerves are abnormally sensitive and send pain messages to the brain on the most minimal stimulation, such as touching. As a result inserting a tampon or intercourse can be extremely uncomfortable or impossible.

Another pattern of vulval pain has been labelled **essential vulvodynia**. This is mainly seen in older or post-menopausal women and is described as an intense burning sensation. The skin looks perfectly normal and is not tender on touching. Again it is now felt that abnormal nerve sensation is in some way responsible for this. Low doses of a type of drug which is normally used to treat depression (tricyclic antidepressants) have helped many of these women.

SORE SEX

Any of the conditions discussed in this chapter may cause problems with a woman's ability to have comfortable and enjoyable sex. In some instances this will be temporary and, as the eczema, or psoriasis or LS improves with treatment, normal sexual activity can be resumed. Sometimes assistance will be needed in terms of discussing variations in sexual positions so that the woman can find a position in which she is most comfortable and in which least irritation occurs. Adequate lubrication is also essential. These aspects should be discussed with your doctor. In addition, specially trained counsellors can help couples to achieve full sexual fulfilment and may be recommended.

VULVAL BIOPSY

In some cases of vulval skin disease a specimen of skin will need to be taken to help with diagnosis or to evaluate a complication of an existing condition. The most uncomfortable part of having a biopsy taken is having the local anaesthetic. This is done with a very fine needle and most patients are unaware of the needle being put in place. The local anaesthetic itself does cause some stinging which lasts for about five to ten seconds. After that, if adequate time is allowed, the rest of the procedure should be painless, although you may be aware of a little bit of tugging in the area. Different doctors finish off the biopsy in different ways. Some prefer to dab on a solution to seal the skin and stop bleeding, while others prefer to put in a stitch. This is usually dissolving and falls out within a week. This is my personal preference as my patients report that they feel more comfortable, more quickly, if they have a stitch as opposed to other methods.

Care of the biopsy site involves gentle salt bathing twice a day until the area becomes comfortable. Once you can touch the area comfortably with your finger it is safe to experiment with resuming sexual activity. By this time you generally have received the results and hopefully things overall are being brought under control.

There are lots of variations on how to have a salt bath. My general instruction is to half-fill a bath with lukewarm water and then add as much salt as can be comfortably held in a closed fist. Making the solution too salty can lead to a bit of burning and irritation. Sit in the bath for five to ten minutes, gently splashing the genital area. If you don't have a bath an appropriate strength of solution can be mixed up by adding a half a teaspoon of salt to a litre of warm water. This is then gently splashed on to the vulva. After either method of application the skin should be dried very gently, either by patting dry with a very soft towel or by using a hair dryer on a cool setting, which sometimes may be more comfortable.

HYGIENE AND THE VULVA

We are often taught that 'squeaky clean' skin is the way to go! In the same way, because the vulva is a moist area where natural fluids are produced and urine and faeces may be present, many women feel that they must apply this 'squeaky clean' philosophy even more strictly to their vulvas. I never cease to be amazed and sometimes horrified by what women do to themselves in the mistaken belief that this is a dirty area. If, in addition, they have problems such as itch or discharge, then they think this means they must be dirty with the result that they clean over-zealously.

Remember:

- In normal women, vaginal secretions contain bacteria which help to protect us from thrush and other infections.

  Douching to remove these has no place in routine daily hygiene and is potentially harmful.

- Vaginal secretions don't build up within the vagina: they constantly, gently seep through the introitus and onto the surface. This not only helps keep the vagina naturally clean, but is important during sexual arousal to make sure lubrication is adequate.

- The tissue of the vestibule is like the tissue of the mouth. You don't wash your mouth out with soap every day, and in the same way you don't need to use soap on the vulva. The vestibule is meant to be moist!

Overcleansing and removing natural secretions from the vulva and vagina not only weaken our natural defences but the products used can be irritants and sometimes contain chemicals which cause allergies. This can result in dermatitis.

The answer is to keep it simple!

Also remember just because something is 'natural' does not make it all right. Soap has a detergent effect whether its ingredients are natural or synthetic. Uranium and cyanide are natural products but that does not make them safe to put on or in our bodies!

Perfumes are a potential source of irritation and allergy— avoid them totally on the vulva. You should particularly steer clear of perfumed products if you have any skin problems and especially if you have a perfume allergy. Many products including toilet papers and sanitary napkins are scented.

Cleansing with water only or salt water is ideal, although many women don't feel clean if they just do this. There are some commercially available cleansing bars and liquids which are soap free and are OK if used sparingly. They are the same as those often recommended by doctors for patients with dry, sensitive skin.

Dry the skin gently. Pat it dry, don't rub.

Underclothes should be loose and absorbent. This is why women with vulval skin problems are advised to wear cotton underwear and avoid stockings or tight jeans and trousers which chafe and make the area warmer and can cause unnecessary rubbing.

If you have a tendency to lose urine when coughing or have other problems with bladder control, this should be reviewed by your doctor. Physiotherapy can be of great benefit. There are a lot of products available now to help women who have problems with bladder control—your pharmacist is generally a good source of information. The products available range from special pads to full underpants with panels into which absorbent materials such as specially designed towlettes or pads can be inserted to give you the strength of protection you need. This will not only help keep your vulva dry and stop irritation caused by your urine, but will also enable you to keep up a healthy social life.

Small amounts of leakage from the anus are not uncommon and this can cause soiling of the underpants and vulva. This is why it is important to wipe yourself from the front to the back after going to the toilet. If the problem is very severe you should have it checked by your doctor.

CONCLUSION

Clearly the vulva is a much more complicated area of our body than we might at first think. It is important that we become familiar with our own bodies and able to express any concerns that we have to our doctors. This is very difficult for many women who may not be used to talking about this area, particularly to a stranger. The simple act of having an examination performed can be very difficult for some women. Some understanding of what can go wrong and the language used will help you deal with such a situation.

The Pap smear is an excellent opportunity for you to raise questions about your sexuality in general or any spot in particular on your vulva that you may be uncertain about. Feeling comfortable with your doctor is very important.

CHAPTER SIX

YOUR CLAWS ARE SHOWING

Nail problems

ANNE HOWARD

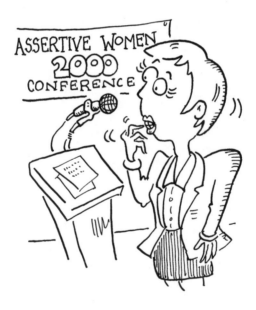

Nails enhance fine touch and dexterity. Healthy shiny nails, perhaps elongated and painted with the help of a good nail manicurist, can make a person feel very sophisticated. Often we just take them for granted. Only when something goes wrong do we start to think about them.

STRUCTURE OF THE NAIL

One of the most important parts of the nail is the **cuticle** (see diagram). It is a small piece of skin that grows down onto the **nail plate** (the hard bit of the nail). It protects the underlying nail **matrix**, which is the tissue from which the nail is formed. If the matrix is damaged by infection or foreign material, the nail plate will become deformed. It is vital therefore not to destroy this cuticle, either by cutting it repeatedly, by pushing it back or even by using cuticle-destroying chemicals.

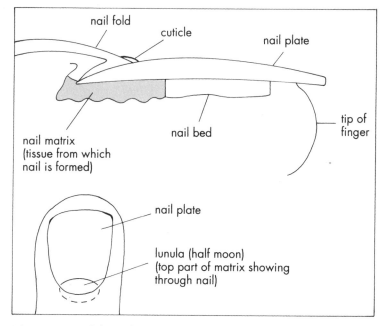

The structure of the nail

The **lunula** is the white half-moon-shaped part of the nail near the cuticle. It is actually the top part of the matrix showing through the nail. Beneath the rest of the nail is the **nail bed** to which the nail plate is firmly attached when the nails are healthy.

BRITTLE NAILS

Brittle and flaking nails are commonly due to contact with harsh soaps and detergents or other irritating substances. This problem is not due to lack of protein, gelatine, calcium or any vitamin. It is very rare for deficiencies of any vitamin or mineral to cause nail problems in our society. In fact, there is not all that much calcium in the nail—its hardness is due to its special protein bonds. Extra protein or gelatine in the diet will not make our nails harder.

When the hands are immersed in water, nail cells swell, then when the nails dry the cells shrink. With repeated swelling and shrinking the nail will eventually split. The best way to prevent your nails from splitting is to keep your hands out of harsh soaps and detergents by wearing water-proof gloves. Cotton-lined gloves or a pair of cotton gloves with rubber or vinyl gloves over these may be necessary to ensure maximum protection.

A coating of clear nail polish, or a nail hardener containing no formalin, will to some extent 'glue' the nail together. Nail polish removers, on the other hand, dry the nail excessively. If you are using polish, a new coat should be applied over the old one in preference to repeatedly removing the old polish with removers. Even nail polish removers labelled 'acetone free' must contain some sort of solvent which, if not acetone, is quite similar to it. Otherwise they would not be able to dissolve the nail varnish.

Nail moisturising creams can help roughness of the surrounding skin but do not penetrate the nail itself. So don't be misled by products whose labels claim that the nails will be nourished or revitalised.

NAILS THAT LIFT

Sometimes the nail plate loses its attachment to the nail bed. The technical term is **onycholysis**. Often there is no obvious cause for this, although again harsh soaps and chemicals are known to contribute to some cases. It is as if the biological glue holding the nail in place fails to do its job. Once the nail is lifted off, infection is likely to occur. Frequently, this is due to the yeast which causes thrush, candida. Sometimes there are bacteria which produce a blue, black or green colour that is very unsightly. This may be mistaken for dirt, but attempts to remove it with a nail file or similar implement will only make the situation worse by forcing the nail even further away from the nail bed.

Likewise attempts to clean out the extra tissue which forms under the lifted nail usually only makes things worse again by damaging the nail bed further. The best thing to do is to keep the nails short, out of water and to blow hot air from a hairdryer underneath several times a day to ensure complete dryness. Sometimes antifungal or antibacterial creams or lotions might be needed. There is no use going on a low-yeast diet. The yeast species in food have nothing to do with the candida species that infects skin. Furthermore if yeast gets under the abnormally elevated nail it gets there from the environment—soil etc.—not via the diet. Infection via foods would imply absorption of the living yeast through the digestive system and into the bloodstream, which is total nonsense!

PARONYCHIA

Paronychia (swollen nail folds) is another problem that occurs more frequently in women and men who habitually immerse their hands in water and/or chemicals which injure that precious piece of skin, the cuticle. Once the cuticle is destroyed the normally sealed and watertight space under the nail fold is open to penetration by moisture. Infection with bacteria and yeasts can then quite easily develop.

If the inflammation goes on long enough, an abnormal ridged and lustreless nail will develop because the accompanying inflammation affects the embryonic nail as it is developing.

People with this problem should wear gloves whenever possible for wet work. Gloves for gardening and even for dirty housework will prevent too much handwashing. Cuticles must *never* be pushed back, cut, or dissolved with chemicals. An antifungal paint applied over the nail fold will stop infection.

In some cases, oral antibiotics or anti-inflammatory creams are needed. Fortunately, paronychia can be cured, although it may take three to six months.

Currently the best available antifungal products are chemicals called imidazoles of which there are a number of brands.

White lines in the nail

Horizontal white lines are common. The appearance is due to part of the nail plate failing to adhere to the bed and is usually the result of some injury, although this may be minor and forgotten. The white lines do not indicate deficiency of vitamins or calcium or any other dietary lack.

Nail biting

The impressive medical term for this common problem is **onychophagia**. It is particularly common in children but many adults are also nail biters. It can lead to stunted and ugly nails. Frequently, bitten and ragged skin along the sides of the nails are associated.

Nail biting does not usually imply nervous problems but is more like a bad habit. There are many suggested 'treatments', for example coating the nails with unpleasant-tasting materials, hypnotism, behavioural therapy, or even bribing!

A fir-tree-like pattern of a longitudinal ridge with grooves on each side can develop in the thumbnails, down the middle of the nail plate. This is due to repeated damage to the middle of the nail fold and is usually a habit problem. People who have this odd nail deformity usually have the habit of repeatedly picking the cuticle with another fingernail.

RIDGED NAILS

As people age, an increased number of longitudinal lines appear in the nails. They are not important and there is no way to prevent them. The nails also become dull and more opaque in old age.

INGROWN TOE NAILS

Some people's big toe nails seem to become increasingly over-curved with time. This is exacerbated by tightly fitting footwear. Overtrimming of the sides of the nail leads to a jagged piece growing into the tissue at the side, which causes inflammation and infection.

Sometimes this can be cured by a change of footwear, correct nail cutting, and inserting a tiny piece of cotton wool under the free edge of the nail to stop it growing into the flesh.

Sometimes surgery is necessary. The surgeon removes the side of the nail right up to and including the matrix so a narrower nail results. This is more comfortable and not particularly unsightly.

FUNGAL INFECTION OF THE NAILS

People prone to tinea of the feet (athlete's foot) sometimes develop this in the nail as well. It is due to a fungus which grows into the nail causing it to become thickened, white or yellow and sometimes crumbly. It can be painful but mainly just looks a bit unsightly. Usually just the toenails, especially the big nails, are involved. Sometimes both toenails and fingernails are infected with the same fungus. People confuse lifted fingernails with fungal infection—the two are quite different. Lifted nails are not in themselves diseased or infected—they have just become unstuck.

Your doctor will need to prescribe tablets to treat the fungal infection, as creams cannot penetrate the nail. Usually you need to be on the tablets for about three months, and it can take a year or more for a new good-looking nail to grow back.

There are, of course, many other causes of crumbly and deformed nails apart from fungal infection and the problems mentioned above. Sometimes the nails are deformed in skin diseases like psoriasis or eczema as well as quite a few other skin conditions. Furthermore, the nails may reflect general health to some degree. Doctors often look at a patient's nails, searching for clues to general health problems like anaemia, some types of lung disease, and circulation diseases.

A major illness or injury sometimes results in a temporary slowing of nail growth, causing odd ridges across the nail to appear a few weeks later. From time to time nail development goes awry during foetal development, resulting in permanent nail deformities for life.

NAIL COSMETICS

Nail polishes

Most polishes contain resins, colouring agents and solvents, giving a shiny appearance and lasting a long time. Some people get an allergic reaction to the resin, oddly enough producing dermatitis on the eyelids rather than around the nail. Low-allergy polishes are available but tend to come off more easily. These days reactions to nail polishes are uncommon. In some situations covering the nail with polish can be a useful way to protect it. Long-term use of coloured polishes often makes the nail yellowish.

Nail polish removers

As far as nail cosmetics are concerned, it is not so much the polish itself but the remover which causes problems.

Removers contain acetone and alcohol, and often damage the surface of the nail, making it lustreless and flaky.

Acrylic nails

There are two main types of artificial nails. The first is a pre-formed synthetic nail which is glued on to the existing nail with an adhesive. The adhesive may provoke an allergic reaction in the skin around the nail, and cause the nail itself to lift off its bed.

The second type of artificial nail is the acrylic nail. A liquid acrylic is mixed with a powder which thickens and is moulded around the natural nail. This hardens quickly to form an artificial nail which is firmly attached to the natural one, and grows out with it. It can be filled in as it grows out. Occasionally severe allergic reactions to the acrylic can occur, resulting in a very damaged nail which takes a long time to return to normal.

CHAPTER SEVEN

WORKING GIRLS

Skin problems in the workplace

ROSEMARY NIXON

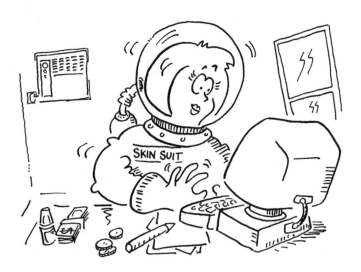

Women have many workplaces: offices, shops, schools, factories, hospitals and, above all, the home.

Skin problems most commonly arise because of contact with an outside agent or substance. Such problems are known as contact dermatitis and, not surprisingly, mainly affect the hands when related to work. Other causes of contact dermatitis may affect other parts of the body, for example the face is often affected when contact dermatitis is related to cosmetics. These will also be considered in this chapter.

About 90 per cent of occupational skin problems are caused by contact dermatitis. Other forms of occupation-related skin disease will also be considered.

CONTACT DERMATITIS

Contact dermatitis can be divided into two types: *irritant contact dermatitis* and *allergic contact dermatitis*.

Irritant contact dermatitis

Irritant contact dermatitis is more common than the allergic type, generally accounting for about 75 per cent of cases. If the stratum corneum (the outer barrier layer) of the skin is visualised as bricks and mortar, then the effect of skin irritants is to destroy the mortar. This then dissolves the stratum corneum and ultimately destroys the whole epidermis (outer skin layer). Initially this causes skin dryness and scaling, but with the triggering of an inflammatory reaction there is progression to redness, itching, and even blistering.

Irritant contact dermatitis may be further sub-divided into *acute* and *chronic* types. Acute irritation usually arises from contact with a single, strong chemical such as a cleaning agent. More common is **chronic** (or *cumulative irritant*) **contact dermatitis**. In this case *repeated* exposure to single or multiple agents combine to damage the skin. These agents can seem innocuous, such as water, soap and detergents, but through their repeated effects on the skin a low-grade irritant contact dermatitis may develop.

Other substances contacted within the home such as laundry detergents, bleach, and sterilising solutions all accentuate the problem. In addition, solvents, oils, greases, dust, fibreglass and wool are all recognised causes of skin irritation. Once dermatitis has occurred, complete recovery may take some time, often months. Even when the hands look normal after an episode of dermatitis, they may take three to four months to recover fully. Until *complete* recovery the skin will remain susceptible to further irritation.

People vary in their susceptibility to skin irritants. Those who are inherently prone to asthma, eczema or hayfever appear to be more susceptible to the development of *irritant* contact dermatitis. In particular, people with a past history of eczema should be warned of the greater risk of developing irritant contact dermatitis if they undertake occupations which involve wet work, for example hairdressing, food preparation, cleaning and mechanical work, particularly when inadequate hand protection is used. Hairdressers especially contact a number of skin irritants such as water, shampoo, and cleaning agents.

Prevention and care

Protection of the hands is the most important way to prevent the development of irritant contact dermatitis. Appropriate gloves should be worn, and they should be discarded if they become torn or if a substance seeps underneath them. While rubber gloves are appropriate for many occupations, it is worth remembering that some chemicals such as solvents will react with rubber, so specific types of gloves may be needed for particular jobs. In addition, it may be useful to wear cotton gloves underneath rubber gloves, particularly in conditions associated with excessive sweating such as when washing dishes in hot water. Otherwise wearing rubber gloves is akin to immersing one's hands in a bag of water!

Once dermatitis has occurred, protection is vital to stop aggravating the condition further. It is often necessary to consult a doctor at this stage for more specific advice on treatment. This may include avoidance of any further contact with skin irritants, even soap. Thus soap substitutes such as pH-balanced mild soaps or emulsifying ointment are often recommended. Moisturising creams, such as 10 per cent glycerine in sorbolene cream, should be applied frequently to reduce the dryness associated with the dermatitis, and can even be applied at night underneath cotton gloves. Finally, topical steroid ointments, applied twice daily sparingly to the actual areas of dermatitis, are often necessary to reduce the skin inflammation.

Other treatments which may be considered include antibiotics for secondary infection and short courses of cortisone tablets in very severe cases. Sometimes specialised light treatment such as PUVA is administered by a dermatologist for conditions that do not respond to other treatments.

The most common occupations for women developing irritant contact dermatitis are hairdressers/beauticians, medical and dental nursing, chefs/butchers/food handlers, cleaners/laundry workers, bar attendant/waitress/kitchen hand. Other occupations which may be associated with problems include laboratory workers, process workers, agriculture/farmer/forest/gardening work, and office work. In men, irritant contact dermatitis is most often seen in those involved with maintenance work, plant operators, fitters and turners, mechanics, engineers, chefs/butchers/food handlers, labourers/trades assistants/process workers, carpenters and woodworkers, and those involved in the construction industry.

Allergic contact dermatitis

Allergic contact dermatitis is less common than irritant contact dermatitis, but can be more severe. It usually starts on the part of the body which is in contact with the **allergen**, that is a chemical which is capable of triggering off the allergic reaction in the skin. Once initiated, the rash can spread widely, either by contact of the chemical with different parts of the body or via a generalised skin reaction in response to the allergen. While the rash may look exactly the same as irritant contact dermatitis with redness and scaling, it is sometimes more severe with weeping and blistering.

Allergic contact dermatitis does not occur after the first episode of skin contact with an allergen. The process of initiating an allergic reaction takes about 7–10 days and thereafter the rash will occur some 4–6 hours after skin contact with the allergen. Interestingly people may become sensitised to an allergen either after the first contact with a chemical, or not for days, months or even years. Women are often amazed when their dermatologist suggests that a cosmetic they have used for years without any problems might be the culprit in the case of a facial rash. The factors which influence a person's likelihood of developing allergic contact dermatitis include their individual susceptibility, the amount and duration of skin contact with the allergen, and also the nature of the allergen itself, some being more likely to cause an allergic reaction.

Testing

Allergic contact dermatitis can be reproduced by clinical testing, traditionally performed by a dermatologist rather than an allergist. This is known as *patch testing*. In patch testing small amounts of chemicals are placed on special hypoallergenic tapes, which are left on the back for two days. The back must be kept dry during this time. The results are read after two days, when the test patches are removed, and then after a further two days. Positive results appear as a red itchy spot, the size of a 5 cent piece. The tests must be performed according to strict international guidelines and in particular it is important to use the correct concentrations of chemicals. This test does not involve pricking the skin and does not test for food allergies or for the type of allergens which might be important in hayfever and asthma, such as pollens, animal products and house dust mite.

If the result is negative, it is important to check that all relevant tests have been performed and nothing has been omitted. It may be that the dermatitis is in fact caused by irritant contact dermatitis, for which there is no actual testing available.

Common triggers

The most common allergen is nickel. People become sensitised to nickel because it is released from costume jewellery which is in close contact with the skin. Nickel allergy is more common in females than males. However, once sensitised, people may react to other sources of nickel in their environment, such as other metallic objects. Fortunately stainless steel objects do not release nickel and do not cause problems. Coins contain nickel however, and cashiers who are sensitive to nickel may develop work-related allergic contact dermatitis. Even gold jewellery may contain a significant amount of nickel and commonly reactions will occur to jewellery which is 9 carat gold. People who are allergic to nickel must use a minimum of 18 carat gold. It is possible to test jewellery for the presence of nickel.

Rubber gloves can cause allergic contact dermatitis, from chemicals known as accelerators which are added to natural rubber during manufacture. Sometimes people develop irritant contact dermatitis as a result of exposure to water and detergents, and then start wearing gloves for the first time. Because the barrier layer of the skin has already been damaged, such people may be more likely to become sensitised to allergens and then develop a secondary rubber allergy as well. Other sources of rubber can also cause problems. These include rubber in footwear, elasticised clothing, tyres, pillows, and even rubber bands. In some cases complicated detective work is needed to pinpoint the cause and to discover the sequence of events which led to the dermatitis!

Chromate is the most common occupational allergen in men, and is found in cement. People who mix bagged cement are particularly at risk of chromate allergy. Cement dust can also irritate the skin, so people may develop a combination of irritant *and* allergic contact dermatitis from working with cement. The allergic reaction may not develop until after many years of working with cement. Chromate is also used to tan leather, and some people react to the small amounts of chromate found in leather, particularly in footwear. This is more likely to occur in cases where there is excessive sweating or if the person is working in a hot environment. Chromate is also used as an anti-corrosive in paints and is used in electroplating, so there are a number of 'at risk' occupations where people might be exposed to this allergen. As a result it may be difficult to avoid.

People may also become allergic to the chemicals used to perm and dye hair. This is mainly a problem for hairdressers who contact such chemicals frequently, although it can rarely also affect the customer. In some instances these chemicals can remain on the hair and continue to cause itchy rashes for days to weeks. It is thus important for hairdressers to protect their hands when handling these chemicals right from the start; otherwise they may develop an allergy which, once triggered, is permanent, even though the rash itself may disappear with time. There is no treatment to get rid of the allergy once it has developed. Desensitisation with regular injections as used for the treatment of pollen and house dust mite allergy is not effective for this type of immunological reaction.

Disinfectants and sterilising agents are often irritating to the skin and can also cause allergy. These may cause problems in hospitals. Glutaraldehyde, for example, is an effective cold sterilising agent used particularly in dental surgeries and to sterilise endoscopy equipment. It may cause a more widespread rash, particularly affecting the face if fumes are present, which is common if the chemical is exposed to the air.

Plants such as primula and alstromeria may cause allergic contact dermatitis in florists who handle them. Rhus and grevillea, in particular the grevillea hybrid 'Robyn Gordon', may also cause rashes. Farmers and outdoor workers, especially in the country may develop Compositae dermatitis. This is an allergic reaction to airborne particles of plants from the chrysanthemum family, particularly capeweed, dogwood and ragweed. It is seasonal, often occurring in spring, and the areas affected tend to be the exposed parts of the face, upper neck, back of hands, and arms.

Specific allergens may be encountered in different jobs, particularly in the manufacturing and construction industries. Epoxy resins are mixed with hardeners to form a resistant coating, or a glue, such as Araldite. Glues may also contain chemicals like acrylates and phenol formaldehyde resins, capable of causing allergic reactions. Wood dusts, for example pine, may cause allergic contact dermatitis because of the presence of a rosin, known as colophony, to which people may react. Colophony is a sticky substance which is responsible for reactions to sticking plaster and adhesive dressings.

People with dermatitis are inclined to use barrier creams and a variety of hand creams, all of which contain preservatives and often fragrances, chemicals which are also capable of causing allergic reactions on the skin.

Of course, it is often necessary to consider *non-occupational* sources of allergens.

Cosmetics contain a variety of chemicals which in some cases will cause allergic reactions. However, *irritant* reactions are again more common than true allergic reactions. People with a history of sensitive skin and especially past eczema are again more susceptible. Sometimes young women in their teens or early 20s who have not had eczema since infancy present with eczema on their eyelids and face which may have been aggravated by use of cosmetics. The presence of *allergic* reactions often needs consideration, however, since identification of the offending allergens through patch testing and their subsequent avoidance may result in complete disappearance of the rash. Allergic reactions often involve the eyelids and neck, since the skin is thinnest on these areas and is thus more sensitive.

The allergens which may need to be considered in cosmetics include fragrance or perfume, lanolin, added sunscreens, emulsifying agents and preservatives such as dowicil (Quaternium 15), imidazolidinyl urea (Germall 115), Kathon CG, formalin, and parabens. Perfume applied directly to the skin often causes rashes. Santalite resin in nail polish classically causes rashes on the eyelids and neck rather than around the fingernails. So-called 'hypoallergenic' cosmetics may contain fewer allergens than others but still need to include preservatives in their formulations and cannot always be relied on as being allergy-free. Similarly, products labelled as 'natural' will often contain fragrances and other chemicals capable of causing allergic reactions. Natural chemicals can cause allergy just as synthetic chemicals can!

The most useful tool for a dermatologist in working out the cause of a facial rash which appears to be an allergic reaction is full ingredient listing on the products. The persistence of Sherlock Holmes is an additional asset!

Finally there is a very long list of chemicals to which dermatologists have seen allergic reactions, although these may be extremely rare. These include reactions to pesticides, paper, clothing dyes, cutting oils and medicaments of all types. There has even been a case of someone with a rash on the buttocks which was traced to an allergy to the varnish on the toilet seat!

Once the offending allergen has been identified and removed, the rash will in many cases disappear. However, in some cases of both irritant and allergic contact dermatitis, the rash is slow to settle, and people who have their rashes for a long time prior to identification and avoidance of the allergen may not improve as readily as those who have had their rashes for only a short time. For this reason early investigation of problems is encouraged.

Some allergens, especially chromate, are notorious for causing persistent rashes despite people avoiding further contact with the chemical. This can lead to a frustrating situation for both patients and doctors. Such problems can only really be solved by preventing the development of the allergy in the first place.

OTHER FORMS OF OCCUPATIONAL SKIN DISEASE

Contact urticaria involves a different type of allergic reaction, known as immediate hypersensitivity—the type of reaction involved in allergy-related hay fever and asthma.

Certain substances trigger immediate reactions when they contact the skin, causing redness and itching within 20 minutes. Typical causes include latex rubber, seafood and vegetables, so this reaction is usually seen in medical or nursing personnel and those working with food, such as chefs. It is tested with 'prick' testing, where small amounts of suspected offending substances are placed onto the forearm skin which is then pricked. A positive reaction is identified as a red wheal which usually occurs within 15 minutes. Very rarely such a reaction can be associated with anaphylaxis, an extremely severe generalised allergic reaction, so this testing must always be done carefully under controlled conditions.

Psoriasis is a relatively common skin condition that may occur where skin is subjected to rubbing or friction. This may be work-related in some cases, for example from handling tools.

Paronychia or nailfold inflammation is occasionally seen in people whose hands are frequently wet. The treatment includes strict avoidance of moisture. (See page 127.)

Infections with fungi, bacteria or viruses may be work-related. Fungal infections are much more common in people working in warm environments. Some forms of fungal infections may be caused by contact with animals. Viral infections which may be work-related include warts in butchers and orf, which can cause large sores on the hands of people in contact with sheep.

Acne can be aggravated by contact with oil or grease and is often worse in the tropics.

Skin cancer may be related to occupational sun exposure. This will be discussed more fully in the next chapter.

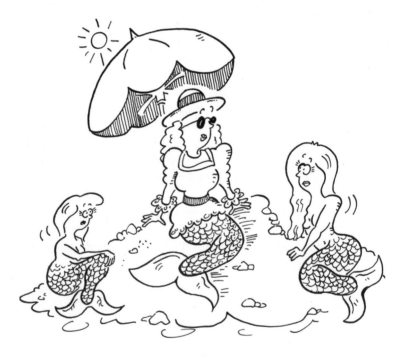

CHAPTER EIGHT

WHY THE SUN IS NOT A GIRL'S BEST FRIEND!

The sun and your skin

ROSEMARY NIXON

Fair-skinned Australians accept many skin changes, such as wrinkles, blotches and spots, as an inevitable part of ageing. The truth is that these changes are related to the time spent in the sun rather than time spent on the planet! This can easily be verified if one compares one's complexion to that of someone of the same age from a less sunny part of the world such as North America or the United Kingdom. An even simpler test is to compare the outer part of one's forearm to the less sun-exposed inner arm.

The many harmful effects of the sun include **sunburn**, the skin changes mentioned above known as **photoageing**, **cataract formation** in the eye and the development of **premalignant lesions** and **malignant skin lesions** (skin cancer). These are balanced only by the pleasurable sensation of warmth which the sun imparts, and the fact that some sun exposure is necessary to form vitamin D in the skin. Nevertheless, recent research has shown that we form enough vitamin D even when using an SPF 15+ screen.

WHAT IS PHOTOAGEING?

Photoageing is a medical term for skin change caused by exposure to ultraviolet light. This includes wrinkling, for example crow's feet, premature ageing of the skin, blotchy blood vessels known as telangiectasia, irregular thinning of the skin, brown spots, furrowing, especially on the back of the neck, and sometimes at a later stage a sallow appearance of the skin.

When normal skin is examined under the microscope the various fibres in the skin's second layer, the dermis, are arranged in an orderly pattern. These fibres give the skin elasticity and resilience. In photoaged skin this orderly pattern is dramatically altered and is replaced by relative chaos. There are clumped abnormal fibres in place of the regular pattern seen in normal skin. This is even observed in the skin of children who have had a degree of sun exposure, although it might be decades before the actual signs are seen on the surface of the skin.

Solar keratoses and **solar lentigines** are common blemishes that occur on photoaged skin.

Solar lentigines, sometimes called 'liver spots', are flat, pale or dark brown spots often found on the backs of the hands or in areas of previous sunburn. They result from an increase in the usual number of pigment-forming cells in the epidermis but they are not pre-malignant or malignant. On the other hand they do occur on sun-damaged skin so are often seen in people who may develop or already have solar keratoses and skin cancers.

Solar keratoses are scaly, often red or pink and sometimes brown, flat or very slightly raised spots which occur on sun-exposed areas such as the face, ears, lower lip, backs of hands, and on bald scalps. Solar keratoses are not skin cancers as such but are pre-malignant lesions. People who develop them have usually had much sun exposure over the years, so may well be at risk of skin cancer. The actual likelihood of malignant change in these is quite low. Solar keratoses are most commonly treated with liquid nitrogen. Other options include the use of an anticancer drug in cream form, 5-fluorouracil, or use of a peeling agent such as salicylic acid in a cream or ointment form.

Bowen's disease spots are slightly larger and pinker than solar keratoses. Women are particularly prone to develop these on the legs, but they can turn up anywhere on the skin, mostly sun-exposed skin. Bowen's disease is technically skin cancer because it is made up of abnormal, malignant cells, but it is *superficial* and not invasive skin cancer. This means that it stays confined to the epidermis, the top layer of skin. On the other hand Bowen's disease spots have a very definite potential to change into invasive skin cancer of the type known as squamous cell carcinoma. They therefore should be removed before this change happens. Appropriate treatments for Bowen's disease are cryosurgery with liquid nitrogen, curettage, or removal by surgical excision.

Liquid nitrogen cryotherapy is a very common treatment for pre-malignant skin spots and superficial skin cancers. It is a very effective treatment because it is extremely cold,

–196°C. Once a lesion is frozen to a temperature of approximately –30°C the tissue dies. The area will then blister and peel off over about a week. After healing there may be a faint white mark due to loss of pigment, especially if the skin is permanently tanned as a result of many years of unprotected sun exposure.

SKIN CANCER

Australia leads the world in the number of skin cancers per head of population. Many fair-skinned people live in the tropical and sub-tropical areas where it is obvious that the original inhabitants of the country have dark, heavily pigmented skin to protect themselves from the sun. The original inhabitants of the other parts of the world traversed by the Tropic of Capricorn or the Tropic of Cancer, such as Africa, South America and Asia, clearly have far more protective skin pigmentation than the people who migrated from western Europe to live in northern Australia.

On the positive side, Australia also leads the world in programs for prevention of skin cancer. While it will be some years before we see all the full benefits of these programs, it has already been established that more and more people are aware of the hazardous effects of the sun and are taking effort and time to slip on protective clothing, slop on some sunscreen and slap on a hat. However, with our extremely high rates of skin cancer we still have a long way to go.

Skin cancer rates have increased over the last 50 to 60 years. This means that Australians were actually developing more skin cancers in the decade *before* sunbathing became a national pastime, which occurred largely in the 1950s. It is not known why skin cancers had already started to increase. Certainly the depletion of the ozone layer may accentuate the problem of skin cancer. It has been estimated that for every 1 per cent decrease in the ozone layer there will be a 2 per cent increase in the amount of harmful ultraviolet light transmitted. UVB is the type of ultraviolet light associated with the development of sunburn and skin cancer.

Basal cell carcinoma

Basal cell carcinoma (BCC) is so called because it develops in the layer of skin called the basal layer where new cells are constantly being formed. Seventy-five per cent of all skin cancers in Australia are of this type. Fortunately it rarely spreads widely to other parts of the body although it does have a propensity to invade into the surrounding skin. In some situations, such as on the face and ear, extensive and disfiguring surgery may be required to remove all the tumour. Dermatologists recognise several different types of BCC by their characteristic appearance and also by where they occur.

Although sun exposure definitely causes BCC, there are other factors which are important. Some people have a genetic predisposition to develop this type of skin cancer. Such people have not had a history of excessive sun exposure in the past. In such cases there is often a history of multiple BCCs in other family members.

Types of basal cell carcinoma

The main types of basal cell carcinomas are the following:

- **Nodulo-ulcerative** is the most common type of BCC and is frequently found on the face. It appears as a skin-coloured lump, often with superficial red blood vessels coursing over the top. It also has a characteristic pearly appearance. It may bleed and develop a central ulcer surrounded by a raised border. **Skin cancers should always be suspected when spots bleed.**
- **Pigmented BCC** are similar to the nodulo-ulcerative type but contain melanin pigment and thus appear black and dark brown. Again they are most commonly found on the face.
- **Morphoeic** (fibrosing) **BCCs** are irregularly shaped, ill-defined plaques which may feel quite firm. This type of BCC spreads in a different way which results in its different appearance. Its edges may be poorly defined, making surgical removal more difficult, and thus these are more likely to recur than the others.

- **Superficial BCCs** are flat, or very slightly raised, red scaly lesions around the size of a 10 cent piece or bigger which occur most commonly on the chest and back. They may look quite similar to Bowen's disease or even like other skin lesions which are not skin cancers, such as psoriasis or eczema. They are very superficial and can be removed by a skin curette, which literally scrapes them off the skin, or by freezing or by excision.

Treatment

The type of treatment chosen as appropriate by your dermatologist will depend on the type and size of the tumour. Sometimes the age and general health of the patient also influences the decision. All treatment methods have a greater than 90 per cent success rate but some tumours will recur in spite of careful removal.

Apart from the treatments mentioned there are other options utilised for special cases. Moh's micrographic surgery is a newly developed technique to remove difficult or large tumours, particularly around the nose and eyes. Interferon is a substance which helps the immune system to combat cancer and has been developed as an injection to treat certain BCCs, although the cure rate is lower.

In some cases even an experienced dermatologist will not be able to diagnose a BCC from its outward appearance and a diagnostic biopsy may be needed. This means removing a small piece of the tumour for examination under the microscope.

In summary BCCs are the most common type of skin cancer, which means they are the most common type of any cancer. Different types of BCC have different appearances and different patterns of growth. Since BCCs rarely spread (metastasise) throughout the body, the main problem with them is that if they are not removed early they can spread locally, ultimately requiring extensive disfiguring surgery. It is important to recognise them before they get to this stage. A skin spot which bleeds may be a BCC!

Squamous cell carcinoma

Squamous cell carcinomas, or SCCs, are so called because they develop from the squamous cells which make up the bulk of the epidermis. They are much less common than BCCs. They occur in older people on sun-exposed sites such as the face, hands, arms and the lower lip. Sometimes they develop in solar keratoses.

People whose immune system is suppressed, for example people with kidney transplants or anyone taking immuno-suppressive drugs, have a higher risk of SCC. Such people are at a much higher risk of skin cancer and must be particularly careful to avoid the sun.

SCCs look like scaly firm lumps on sun-exposed areas. Sometimes these are quite tender. Bleeding and ulceration may occur, although less commonly than with BCCs. The risk of spread throughout the body is about 2 per cent, but is more likely to occur for those on the lower lip and ear. Thus these lesions should be treated as soon as possible.

The appropriate treatment of SCCs is surgical removal. Occasionally, especially in the elderly, treatment with radio-therapy rather than surgery may be appropriate.

Malignant melanoma

Melanoma is a malignant tumour of the pigment-forming cells of the skin, the melanocytes. Fortunately malignant melanoma is far less common than BCCs and SCCs, which are termed non-melanocytic skin cancers. The incidence of melanoma has been estimated at approximately 20–60 cases per 100 000 people, depending on where people live. Queensland has the highest rate of melanoma in the world.

Melanoma have the ability to spread throughout the body making them the most deadly form of skin cancer. Approximately 5–10 per cent of people who have this skin cancer will die as a result of it, but fortunately this percentage is becoming smaller because dermatologists are now able to recognise the very early and subtle changes in moles which might signal the start of a melanoma. If a melanoma is removed in the early stages then the risk of dying from it is extremely low.

Melanomas are becoming more and more common and the reasons for this are not yet clear. Statistics show that the increase in melanoma preceded the fashion for skin tanning.

Dermatologists recognise several risk factors for melanoma. Although the sun clearly plays a role, the actual mechanism has not been established. The incidence of melanoma is inversely related to latitude, that is, people living closer to the Equator in Queensland have a much higher rate than people living in Victoria. The same relationship has been established in the USA but does not fit in Europe where people living closer to the equator have more skin pigmentation. It has been assumed that the relationship between melanoma with latitude reflects increased sun exposure or increased time spent outside.

People more likely to develop melanoma are those with large numbers of moles (**naevi**) and those who burn easily and tan poorly. People who have had excessive, intermittent sun exposure producing sunburns are also thought to be at increased risk. Statistics also show that family members of people with melanomas have an increased risk of developing melanomas themselves. People who work *inside* are slightly more at risk for melanoma than *outdoor* workers, a surprising finding! The explanation for this may be that people who work indoors are more likely to organise the sort of holidays where they are likely to have intense sun exposure.

Types of malignant melanoma

Dermatologists recognise different types of melanoma.

- **Superficial spreading melanoma** is the most common melanoma, and especially affects people in the 30 to 60 year age bracket. Males tend to develop them on the back and chest, whereas females tend to develop them on their legs. The most striking feature is irregular pigmentation. They usually show a mixture of colours varying from black or dark brown to red or pink. They usually have an irregular outline and are often flat, although they may become raised later on. They are usually 6–7 mm in diameter, but dermatologists are increasingly picking up early and even smaller melanomas. There may be absolutely no symptoms associated with this skin cancer, although in the later stages bleeding and itching may occur. It is most important therefore that people *look* at their skin regularly with good lighting, since these melanomas are not felt on touching the skin and may otherwise be easily ignored.

- **Nodular melanomas** affect a slightly older age group, with a slight male predominance. They are mostly black or dark blue lumps which often grow rapidly. They have a tendency to ulcerate and bleed.
- **Lentigo maligna melanomas** affect the elderly, with equal incidence in males and females. They most commonly occur on the head and neck. Often prior to the development of the melanoma, there is a long history of a flat brown spot on the face known as a Hutchinson's melanotic freckle, also called lentigo maligna. When melanoma develops there is usually irregular pigmentation, often with dark areas and an irregular border, and sometimes raised areas. These melanomas occur in people with high lifetime sun exposure.
- **Acral lentiginous melanomas** occur on the hands, feet and around the nails and are more common in some racial groups, particularly Asians. They are not very common in Caucasians.

Melanomas may less commonly affect the conjunctivae, which is the membrane covering the outer lining of the eye, the lining of the mouth, and the vulva. Women should self-examine the vulva or have it checked for unusual moles and pigmentation when their yearly pap smear is done.

Warning signs of melanoma

(i) The development of irregular colour in a skin lesion, which may either be a pre-existing mole *or* a new spot.

(ii) The development of an irregular edge or border.

(iii) Increase in size or sudden appearance of a mole or freckle.

(iv) Symptoms such as itching, bleeding, lumpiness or any change in a mole or freckle.

Prognosis of malignant melanoma

Five factors are important for the longterm outlook (prognosis) in an individual patient with melanoma:

(i) *Thickness of the melanoma*. The thinner melanomas are, the better the prognosis is. People who collect cancer statistics talk about five year survival, which literally means the percentage of people who have not died five years after the cancer has been removed. People whose melanomas were very thin (less than 0.76 mm) when removed have a 98% chance of still being alive five years later. The survival rate drops to around 45% for people with melanomas more than 4 mm thick.

(ii) *Level*. The level in the skin to which the melanoma grows is thought to give a good indication of the biological properties of the tumour. Level 1 means that the malignant cells are confined to the epidermis and thus have not invaded at all, and once these are removed they are completely cured. Level 2 means that the malignant cells have grown to the very top part of the dermis. Levels 3, 4 and 5 indicate progressively deeper levels of growth. The histopathologist who examines the biopsy will report on the level of tumour spread.

(iii) *Location*. In terms of likelihood of spread to the rest of the body, the worst areas to have a melanoma are the head, neck and back. This is thought to represent the greater ease with which the melanoma may spread throughout the body.

(iv) *Sex*. Statistics show that females have a better prognosis than males.

(v) *Ulceration*. If a melanoma becomes ulcerated it usually means that there is a higher likelihood that the tumour cells have already spread to other parts of the body.

How are melanomas treated?

The most important aspect of treating melanoma is to diagnose it as early as possible and to remove it completely. Melanomas must be removed before they spread throughout the body. Once they do spread none of the current treatments available is effective, although there are many new treatments, including melanoma vaccines, being tested. A suspected melanoma must be removed, ideally in its entirety, so the whole lesion can be examined by a histopathologist and the diagnosis confirmed as well as the level and thickness established. Based on this information it may be decided to take extra skin from the initial site of the melanoma. This area around the melanoma is at higher risk of the tumour recurring, but removal of extra skin from the site does not actually affect the final outcome. This means it is rarely necessary to resort to drastic surgical measures to achieve the best possible prognosis. However there are some instances where further surgical treatment is recommended, such as removing lymph glands.

Following removal of the tumour it is important that patients are examined in order to discover any changes in lymph glands which may indicate recurrence of the melanoma. People with one melanoma are at increased risk of developing another melanoma, so the rest of their skin should be checked yearly. Finally, family members should also be warned that they too have a slightly increased risk of melanoma.

BENIGN SKIN LESIONS

Moles, or **naevi,** are collections of pigment cells within the skin. Various types are recognised based largely on where they are positioned in the two layers of the skin, the epidermis and dermis.

Junctional naevi are so called because the cells of which they are composed are situated at the junction of the epidermis and dermis. They are flat, mid to dark brown moles which first appear in childhood. The number of potential moles an individual has seems to be genetically predetermined, but it also seems that sun exposure provokes their actual appearance on the skin.

It is not necessary to have all your junctional naevi removed. In the main they are harmless blemishes, although it is recognised that they have some potential to develop into melanoma. It should be stressed that this risk of conversion to melanoma is extremely low. It is certainly not appropriate —or practical—to remove all these moles just because of the very small risk, especially as we know that melanomas also develop in normal skin and not only in moles.

Compound naevi are moles in which the pigmented cells are located at the junction of the epidermis and dermis and also in the dermis. Thus these often have a two-tone character with a raised central area, the part in the dermis, and a surrounding flat area, the part at the junction. When the component in the dermis matures, which it may do with time, people may notice that the mole is becoming raised. This often prompts them to see their doctor to have the moles checked. Such a check is wise, although the change is not a sign of melanoma in this case.

In **intradermal naevi**, all the pigmented cells are situated in the dermis. They have lost their potential to change and are totally benign moles. With time they may lose their colour, and become soft like skin tags. Treatment is only required for cosmetic reasons if desired by the patient.

Dysplastic naevi are junctional or compound naevi which have some irregular features, both on the surface of the skin and on examination under the microscope. Many people just have one or two dysplastic naevi and this is not associated with an increased risk of melanoma. However, there is a very rare situation in which virtually all family members have many dysplastic naevi and these people have a very high risk of melanoma. People who have a few dysplastic naevi are often photographed and checked regularly to make sure that melanoma does not develop in any of their moles. It is not appropriate to remove all the moles because melanomas more often arise in normal skin, as mentioned above.

It takes training and experience to be able to distinguish one type of mole from another. If you have any concerns about your moles it is worth asking your doctor or dermatologist for advice—it beats worrying unnecessarily!

KEEPING OUT OF THE SUN

It is the ultraviolet B component of sunlight that is the most harmful, particularly in the causation of sunburn and skin cancer. Usually UVB is principally found in the midday summer sun, and hence protection from the sun is advised between the hours of 10 a.m. and 2 p.m., or 11 a.m. and 3 p.m. with daylight saving. You should observe a 'solar curfew' at this time, if possible. Maximal amounts of UVB occur in mid summer.

The factors which influence the amount of UVB reaching the earth include:
(i)   altitude
(ii) scattering by atmospheric molecules, particles and water droplets (clouds)
(iii) reflection from surfaces such as snow, sand and water.

In high altitudes there will be an increasing amount of ultraviolet light, with a 20 per cent increase at 1500 m. Skiers are well aware of the increased possibility of sunburn, especially on clear sunny days!

Atmospheric particles will influence the amount of ultraviolet light but it is important to recognise that significant amounts of UVB can still occur even when there is some cloud cover or on hazy days.

Reflection is especially important from surfaces like sand and water. This is most apparent when people protect themselves from direct sunlight with the use of hats or beach umbrellas, but still burn because of reflected ultraviolet light.

Note that temperature is not mentioned. Ultraviolet light is neither hot nor cold. Days of 20°C can be associated with as much UVB exposure as days of 35°C. This fact is easily appreciated by observing charts of UVB measurements which are included on the weather reports in summer in Australia. Irrespective of the daily temperature there is an increase in UVB in the middle of the day, although there is some variation in the absolute level reached. In the past, people used the term windburn to denote sunburn occurring on cool or cloudy days. In fact there is no such thing as windburn. It is just sunburn.

The principles of sun protection are as follows:

a   *Avoid* unnecessary sun exposure between 10 a.m. and 3 p.m.
b   *Block* effects of sunlight with protective clothing, wide-brimmed hats, and sunglasses
c   *Cover* up with sunscreens
d   *Do not* sunbathe or use solar lamps
e   *Educate* children.

Sunscreens

Sunscreens may be comprised of chemical blocking agents which absorb UV light or physical blocking agents such as titanium dioxide or a combination of both. The base may be alcohol, a water or oil-based lotion, an ointment or a cream.

The sun protection factor, SPF, is the ratio of the dose of UV needed to produce burning *with* the sunscreen on the skin to the UV dose needed to produce the same amount of burning *without* sunscreen on the skin. For example, if it normally takes you 10 minutes to burn then theoretically an SPF of 15 allows you to stay in the sun 15×10 minutes before getting sunburnt. After this time the skin will have been exposed to as much sun as it can handle, so that this period should *not* be extended. The Australasian College of Dermatologists in its consensus statement on photoageing and Photodamage states: 'The use of sunscreens to extend sun exposure time negates the beneficial effects of these agents' (*Photoaging & Photodamage as a Public Health Concern*. The Australasian College of Dermatologists Consensus Statement 1989). It is true that sunscreen often needs to be applied more frequently because of sweating and swimming which wash it away from the skin. While sunscreens labelled with SPF values greater than 15 are available overseas, it can be seen from the following table that there is little additional benefit at the higher SPF values. In fact adverse reactions are more likely with increasing concentrations of sunscreening chemicals.

Sun protection factor	Percentage reduction of UVB
2	50%
4	75%
8	87.5%
16	93.8%
32	96.9%

Sunscreen containing chemical sunscreening agents should be applied 15–20 minutes prior to going out in the sun so that the chemicals can bind with the outer layer of the skin.

Sunscreens not uncommonly cause irritation of the skin, but true allergic reactions are uncommon. Most problems relate to the fact that these products are often applied in hot conditions when sweating is likely. People prone to eczema or with sensitive skin are more likely to develop skin irritation.

Exposure during work can be an important contributing factor in the development of skin cancer. It is appropriate that work duties and leisure pursuits be organised to avoid sun exposure during the middle of the day. Protective measures such as clothing and sunscreens are also very important. Sunscreens should be applied not only to the face but *also* the back of the hands, back of the neck, ears, lips, particularly the lower lip, and bald scalps. These are the areas where skin cancers most commonly develop.

A word about solariums

The Anti-Cancer Council and the Australasian College of Dermatologists warn that the use of solariums is not safe. While these have tended to use UVA rather than the more harmful UVB, UVA may also play a role in causing skin cancer. UVA penetrates more deeply into the skin and it certainly contributes to photoageing. Finally, small amounts of UVB may be produced by these machines. Not only can this give rise to skin cancers but also to cataract formation in the eye.

In summary a tan is a sign of skin damage! Over recent years even the models in glossy magazines have become paler and even the cosmetic companies are beginning to promote fair skin as more fashionable. *There is no such thing as a healthy tan!*

CHAPTER NINE

IMPROVING ON NATURE

What you can do to improve your skin

BARBARA BREADON

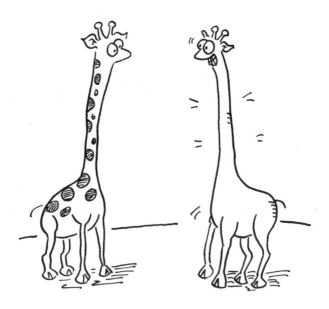

Despite all the advertising implying the contrary, the type of skin you have is largely inherited. If you are genetically lucky and have inherited good skin, there is very little you can do to ruin it—apart from basking in the sun, of course! If you are not so lucky, there are no creams, poultices, potions, ampoules or unguents which will change the basic *quality* of your skin. Advertised elixirs of youth and beauty are misleading and the benefits illusory. All is not lost, however! You may be stuck with the type of skin you have inherited but if you are not satisfied with it there *are* ways to improve on nature.

How to make the most of what you've got

Take home renovation as an analogy. A house with building faults or suffering bad structural damage as a result of collapsed foundations needs restumping or reblocking. In other words, it needs major repair work. Likewise, if your face has structural defects either from birth or due to injury, or if the facial muscles and tissues are sagging as a result of ageing and photoageing (sun damage) you may choose to consult a plastic surgeon. Plastic surgery can now offer face and brow lifts, and contouring and resurfacing techniques of various kinds. It is possible to have noses remodelled so that the shape is entirely changed, eyes can be altered in shape, eyebrows elevated, bags under the eyes removed, lips made fuller, and even cheekbones made more prominent. Fat deposits can be removed by liposuction and hair can be transplanted. Most of these procedures are relatively major and certainly carry risks—as with any surgical procedure. Make sure the person who treats you has the appropriate specialist qualifications. Any doctor can call herself or himself a cosmetic surgeon but only those with extensive training can call themselves plastic surgeons.

If the problem is with the *quality* of the skin itself, whether its colour, texture or the presence of various blotches and blemishes, a dermatologist can help using a variety of techniques which really *can* improve on nature. This particularly applies to aged and photoaged skin.

Cosmetic camouflage is one option. A good cosmetic artist can teach the skills necessary to apply cosmetics correctly. Many blemishes can be hidden with 'paint and paper'. This particularly applies to major blemishes due to malformations or birthmarks (port wine stains and others, see chapter 1). Removal of the offending blemishes is another option. There are various techniques available for removing excrescences, irregular pigmentation and eliminating so-called broken blood vessels. *Contour* can be improved with filling agents such as collagen. *Texture* can be improved by various peeling or resurfacing techniques.

Few of the above renovations would be necessary if we all adopted strict sun-protective measures from infancy. Alas, it is too late for some of us, but our children and our children's children should benefit from what we now know about sun exposure and its effect on the skin.

HOW TO CARE FOR YOUR SKIN

Many advertising dollars are spent on making us feel guilty if we do not follow a regime of skin care. However in the case of skin, *less is more*. The exhortation to 'cleanse, tone, nourish and revitalise' is a catchcry designed to maintain the health of the cosmetic industry, not your skin.

If you are concerned about your own health, the next time you are tempted to buy an expensive elixir of youth in a jar, think again. Spend the money instead on sunscreen, and see your doctor for a mole check, learn breast self-examination, and have a pap smear. You will still have enough money left to donate to your favourite charity, enjoy coffee with friends, and feel a warm inner glow.

Cleansing and maintenance

We clean our skin to remove the surface film of grime, dead skin cells and applied cosmetics mingled with sebum and sweat. The most effective way to do this is with soap and water, which is cheap and usually readily available. Soap and water are more effective than water alone as soap has a degreasing action; it dissolves the surface grease. Of course we are not trying to achieve 'brighter than bright' or 'cleaner than clean', so use a soap that is mild and non-irritating. If the skin is stripped of too much natural grease, the surface begins to flake and redden. Natural skin oil is produced for a purpose: it lubricates our skin surface and helps provide a barrier against irritating substances from the outside environment.

Cleansing creams and lotions range from thicker water-in-oil types to more fluid oil-in-water types. They work by blending with the surface grime and debris (including dead surface cells), which can then be wiped or rinsed off. These may be used for cleaning the skin but are no more efficient than soap and water. In addition, they can leave a residue which may encourage pores to block and lead to blackheads. Acne sufferers should be especially wary of these products.

Astringents, often called toners or fresheners, are not recommended by dermatologists. These are based on alcohol, which is a solvent. Their use is *not* an essential part of skin care, as is often implied. They are simply degreasing agents and impart a pleasant tingle as the alcohol evaporates and cools the skin. They do *not* close pores as is often claimed. Apart from a possible psychological benefit, there is no advantage to be gained from using toners. Only use toners if you enjoy the feeling, provided you do not have dry skin as the alcohol will certainly add to the dryness.

Scrubs and exfoliating creams are often promoted as a superior method of cleaning the skin but they have no special usefulness for normal skin and are capable of making the skin irritated and dry. In any case, our skin exfoliates naturally without the need for extra help as we are constantly shedding dead surface cells in the form of minute invisible skin flakes. Sun-damaged skin may benefit from some types of peeling creams or lotions (see page 169).

Moisturising the skin

Moisturisers lubricate the skin but are only necessary if your skin is dry. This applies to approximately one in ten people. Alternative names used by the beauty industry include emollient, humectant, nourishing cream, skin food, firming lotion and anti-wrinkle cream. These glamorous names imply superior properties which these creams simply do not possess.

Moisturisers merely put a film of oil on the skin surface, which in turn seals in moisture and prevents water loss from the outer layers of skin through evaporation. They also smooth down surface scale, giving the skin a more supple feel and smoother appearance, so that if your skin is slightly flaky, applying a moisturiser can make the skin appear more normal.

Water loss from the outer skin layers is more likely to occur in dry climates with low humidity, particularly in cold winter weather and centrally-heated or air-conditioned interiors. You may notice increased dryness and even flakiness of the skin in these situations. Moisturisers only seal in the natural water content of our skin, which comes from the blood supply and sweat glands. Water cannot be added to your skin by splashing on tap water or spraying on mineral water. Likewise, moisturisers cannot penetrate the living cell layers of the epidermis. The skin's nourishment comes from its blood supply, a rich network of capillaries just under the epidermis. It is total nonsense to talk of nourishing creams and skin foods.

The proportion of oil and water in different moisturisers and preparations varies, hence their different properties. More greasy preparations are often promoted as night cream or nourishing cream, whereas non-greasy types are often promoted as vanishing cream or day cream to be used under make-up. Moisturisers do not prevent wrinkles or ageing despite claims to the contrary. Wrinkles are caused by structural changes in the skin as a natural part of skin ageing. They are exaggerated and accelerated by sun exposure. The oils in moisturisers cannot penetrate through the layers of the epidermis to a level where wrinkles are formed. Even if this were possible, they could not be incorporated into the skin's biological structure.

Various ingredients added to moisturisers have been promoted as breakthroughs and claimed to repair DNA, prevent wrinkling, reverse sun damage, promote cell regeneration, repair collagen and improve tone. Such added ingredients include protein, vitamins, collagen, elastin, hormones, aloe vera, placental extract and a host of other substances. All these come with a hefty price tag, but simple cheap preparations which you can buy from your chemist or supermarket work just as well as any other moisturiser.

Beware of pseudoscientific jargon. If something comes in an ampoule it does not necessarily mean that it will work any differently from a product that comes in a jar or tube, although it will most likely cost more. Price is no guarantee of quality. You are paying for the advertising, packaging and image. Other traps include the promotion of products as 'natural', 'organic' or 'herbal', thereby implying superiority. All creams and cosmetics need preservatives to prevent deterioration and therefore must contain chemicals.

Let's face it, water is a chemical (H_2O) and we humans are 70 per cent water with the addition of a pot-pourri of other chemicals including proteins, amino acids and fats. Terms such as 'natural' and 'organic' are misleading to say the least. Likewise, words such as 'dermatologist tested' do not ensure quality. This type of trendy labelling is simply designed to produce a sense of security in the customer. Details of scientific studies are carefully withheld. No one tells you which medical journal published the conclusions of these studies or whether they were published at all. There is no reason why a face cream 'researched in a Swiss clinic' or 'used by millions of French women' should be any different from one made in Australia, although some women may think this sounds more glamorous. So maintain a healthy scepticism when buying cosmetic products. Beware of the promotion of creams for specific areas of skin or times of day. We do not need eye, neck and throat creams, or special creams for day and night. We merely need moisturisers to correct dryness (if present) on any area at any time. Legislation is planned which will curb the extravagance of cosmetic advertising and severely limit the types of statements that can be made.

'Hypoallergenic' is a trendy term which is basically meaningless and usually indicates that no perfume has been added to the product. Most cosmetics contain dozens of different ingredients and some of these can cause allergic reactions in certain people. Some people are allergic to the preservatives or sunscreens incorporated into cosmetic products, so just leaving out the perfume cannot guarantee that a product will not cause an allergic reaction.

Masks and facials

Masks fall into the category of pampering. As long as it does not irritate your skin a mask might make your skin feel temporarily fresher and smoother. Some masks are just mixtures of various moisturisers that come with instructions to apply, leave on for twenty minutes, then rinse off. Others are clay-based. These harden as they dry on the skin (egg white does the same) so that the skin can temporarily look more taut. They also impart a pleasant tingling sensation as a result of a mild irritant effect on the skin. Clay masks may also make the skin look temporarily less oily. Whatever they claim to do, they are in contact with the skin for a very short time so any effect is short-lived. Clay masks are also capable of producing dryness and irritation, particularly if left on for too long.

Facials certainly fall into the pampering and 'feel good' category. If you wish to pay for someone to clean your skin with 'cleansing cream', massage your face with moisturisers and perhaps apply a mask, go ahead, provided your skin is normal and you can afford it. It certainly can be a pleasant way to spend an hour and there is no doubt that many beauticians are extremely skilled in giving facials so that one can emerge feeling quite relaxed. You should be alert to the fact that the impressive-looking instruments used by beauticians are simply devices for massaging the skin or for giving small electric impulses. This causes the skin to temporarily flush and swell, so that fine lines look less obvious for a very short while. Other devices are used to steam the skin, and give the same effect.

On the subject of steaming, it is true that pre-steaming may make blackheads easier to squeeze out because the skin around the opening of the blackhead is softened by the water and heat. It will not help deep-seated acne pimples. In fact, facials may cause problems in acne-prone skin because the oily moisturisers and cleansing creams used can encourage pores to clog and blackheads to form.

USE OF COSMETICS TO IMPROVE ON NATURE

Cosmetics are used (and have been for thousands of years) to improve on nature by either camouflaging minor blemishes or adding colour. As such, they can definitely improve the appearance. It is equally true that great skin can look good without any cosmetics.

As long as we have a multi-million dollar cosmetics industry, the completely natural look will probably never be popular. Cosmetics also have a protective function. Moisturising types act like any moisturiser to seal in water and prevent water loss by evaporation. Opaque foundations contain titanium dioxide which reflects harmful ultraviolet rays and others contain chemical sunscreens which filter out ultraviolet rays.

The foundation you choose depends on your skin type and colour. For example, those with acne and oily skin should avoid oil-based foundations. If your skin is dry, use a creamier or oilier product. Foundation should be thoroughly washed off before going to bed to prevent it building up on the skin, leading to pores clogging and blackheads forming.

Powder is the finishing touch to give a matt smooth appearance and create a more even look. Powders can be coloured or translucent. The basic ingredient is talc, which also absorbs oil and helps promote the matt look. It is personal choice as to whether you use loose or pressed powder. In general, powder causes few problems with allergic or irritant reactions.

Lipstick helps to protect the lips by absorbing ultraviolet rays. The darker the colour, the better the protection. Some lipsticks have chemical sunscreens included, which add to the protection.

Eyeshadow, mascara and eyeliner can certainly improve the appearance of the eyes. Allergic and irritant reactions can occur and, for this reason, products need to be tested carefully to ensure they do not irritate the skin around the eyes. Eyelid skin is thinner and more vulnerable than other facial skin and is therefore more prone to dermatitis. Oddly enough, the most common causes of eyelid dermatitis are nail cosmetics and volatile substances like perfumes and hair sprays. It is amazing how often we touch our eyes during the day. Eyebrow and eyelash dyes can definitely cause allergic reactions and should be approached very cautiously. A note of caution has also been sounded about tattooing to create a permanent eyebrow or eyeline, as some allergic and scar-like reactions have developed. Eyeshadows are particularly likely to cause problems as they are applied to the most vulnerable part of the thin skin of the eyelids.

Frosted eyeshadows contain ground-up fish scales or mica to produce their iridescent appearance. It is not surprising that they cause irritation.

Camouflage make-up

Special cosmetics can help camouflage various types of birthmarks, especially the ones consisting of dilated capillaries (for example, port wine stains, see chapter 1) and large pigmented birthmarks. Your dermatologist can give advice on the types of cosmetics available. It is certainly worthwhile consulting someone with the expertise to teach you how to apply such cosmetics for maximum effect and help you choose a shade appropriate for the blemish. A good camouflage make-up needs to be water-resistant to allow swimming, and it must not be easily rubbed off or affected by sweating.

Not all blemishes that need camouflage occur on the face. Scars from burns, surgery, accidents, some acne and radiotherapy anywhere on the body can all be camouflaged.

Women with ruddy complexions or dilated capillaries on their faces ('broken capillaries') may benefit from using a foundation that absorbs light in the red spectrum. This is why green-tinted foundations are usually recommended. White or 'pearlescent' foundations recommended by many cosmetic companies are also useful for camouflaging broken capillaries and brown spots.

Out, damned spot!

Some harmless but unattractive blemishes tend to appear on our skin as we age. The most common are seborrhoeic keratoses (also known as seborrhoeic warts and sometimes unflatteringly alluded to as senile warts). These usually appear as raised, rough warty growths which vary in colour from flesh-coloured or pink through to greyish brown and even black. The surface texture ranges from smooth to scaly and rough. Seborrhoeic warts appear on the trunk, face and neck, and are more common in middle age. One particularly annoying variety takes the form of skin tags which often grow on the neck, armpits and groin. The larger types are more common in overweight people. Seborrhoeic keratoses are not skin cancers but dermatologists are often asked to remove them for cosmetic reasons. They are removed by either burning them with a fine electric needle (diathermy or cautery), scraping them off with a skin curette, or freezing them (cryotherapy).

'Liver spots' (nothing to do with the liver) or 'age spots' result from skin ageing and sun exposure and occur on sun-exposed skin, especially the hands and face. They look like large, irregular freckles. They can be faded with light cautery or freezing and some forms of laser. Bleaching creams containing hydroquinone can be used to improve results after treatments but these must be used carefully and under medical supervision as some can cause irritation.

Sun-damaged skin of the face is prone to develop blackheads and small oil cysts (whiteheads). These come about because of sun-induced degeneration of the elastic tissue in the skin. These tiny cysts can be painstakingly removed using minute incisions. They cannot be squeezed out. Another frequent occurrence in ageing skin is the appearance of overgrown sebaceous glands (sebaceous adenomata) which appear as yellowish clumps of tissue, mainly on the forehead and temple area. They are sometimes mistaken for skin cancers (BCCs). The only successful method of removing these entirely is surgical excision, or cautery if they are small.

WHAT CAN WE REALLY DO FOR AGEING SKIN?

First we need to know what happens when our skin ages. Most skin ageing is photoageing. In other words, it is due to sun damage acquired throughout life. On your own body you can easily see the effect of photoageing if you compare exposed to adjacent non-exposed areas, e.g. buttock or breast skin with nearby leg or chest skin that has had more sun exposure. Chronic sun damage probably accounts for 80–90 per cent of the changes we associate with ageing of the skin. These include dryness and flakiness, irregular pigmentation, fine crisscross wrinkling, broken capillaries, sallowness, and a general coarsening of the skin. Of course skin, like any other body organ, ages chronologically—it deteriorates as our bodies grow older—so the skin of a person over 50, even on areas never exposed to the sun, will be different from the skin of a young child.

The epidermis (our skin's top layer) becomes thinner as we age. At the same time, the outermost layer of the epidermis (the stratum corneum) thickens in some areas with the result that older skins often look drier and more flaky. The oil and sweat glands are also less active in old age and this contributes to the dryness. Another part of normal ageing are the expression lines on the face from muscle activity. These include frown lines on the forehead, laughter lines (crow's feet) at the corners of the eyes, and 'purse string' lines around the mouth. Fat is deposited in certain areas of the face (and body!) as we age and muscle tone decreases. Add to this the effects of gravity causing tissues to sag, and the end result is jowls, bags under the eyes and loose skin under the chin (dewlap). Sometimes grooves develop on the face as a result of an habitual sleeping position.

Elastin and collagen are special fibres in the dermis (the layer under the epidermis) which give the skin elasticity and suppleness as well as strength and resilience. Sun damage over a lifetime causes the fibres to degenerate, become clumped and lose their orderly arrangement. These changes are referred to in medical jargon as **solar elastosis**. Solar elastosis contributes to the fine crisscross wrinkling of photoaged skin. In such skin the expression-line type of wrinkling is more exaggerated. This is also more marked in the skin of smokers.

DNA is less likely to repair itself correctly, leading to mistakes in cell division that result in the likelihood of tumours and the development of abnormal cells. This is the reason that photoaged skin is prone to solar keratoses and skin cancers. Pigment cells often wear out and fail to produce any colour at all, causing white spots on the skin—very common on the forearms and lower legs. Another result of sun damage is that your skin does not tan so easily or evenly as you age. In other areas the pigment cells produce too much pigment and the result is solar lentigines or 'age spots'. The capillary networks just below the epidermis dilate and become more prominent because they are not as well supported by the degenerated elastic tissue.

In the real world, the most conscientious use of sun protection will not totally prevent sun damage. After all, most of us enjoy being outdoors occasionally. Although we can do little to stop chronological ageing, our skin will stay younger-looking for a lot longer if sun protection is practised from infancy.

WHAT CAN WE DO IF PHOTOAGEING IS ALREADY PRESENT?

Two substances have been endorsed by dermatologists to date as possibly improving some of the signs of sun damage. Neither is a magic potion or a fountain of youth. One is tretinoin or retinoic acid. The other is glycolic acid, which is used as a light peeling agent to improve the appearance of sun-damaged skin.

Tretinoin is a medication that was primarily used to treat acne (see chapter 2). It is a synthetic chemical based on vitamin

A. In addition to inducing a mild surface peeling, thereby removing dead surface cells, tretinoin may improve the quality of collagen in the dermis. Used regularly over several months, it may improve *some* of the unpleasant changes due to photoageing. Tretinoin will help the very fine wrinkling, blotchy freckling, and scaly patches associated with sun damage. It will not reverse or remove wrinkles and expression lines caused by muscle movement and gravity. It will not remove broken capillaries, and may make them worse by causing irritation and reddening of the skin. It is not a wonder treatment and needs to be persevered with for about twelve months before you will see an improvement. It needs to be continued intermittently for life to maintain the improvement, and must always be combined with strict sun protection measures.

Tretinoin cream should be applied at night about twenty to thirty minutes after washing your face with mild soap and water. As well as the face, it can be used on the neck, upper chest and forearms, and even the hands, or anywhere skin is sun damaged. You should avoid applying it very close to the eyes and mouth where irritation is more likely to occur.

The main side effect is skin irritation causing the skin to become red, dry and flaky. There may be slight itching or a burning sensation. This affects different people to different degrees. It can be minimised by starting slowly, using the cream every second or third night for the first few weeks and gradually building up the frequency of applications as your skin becomes used to the cream. Tretinoin cream also makes your skin more sensitive to the sun so that you are more likely to sunburn in the areas where it has been applied. It is therefore important to use an SPF 15+ sunscreen regularly (ideally, every day) even during winter.

Tretinoin cream should not be used during pregnancy (chemicals of this class, known as retinoid drugs, are known to cause damage to the developing foetus).

Glycolic acid is one of the 'fruit acids'. These include citric acid (in citrus fruits), malic acid (found in apples) and lactic acid (found in milk). When applied to the skin, glycolic acid loosens the cells which make up the top layer of the epidermis and induces peeling. The degree of peeling depends on the strength of the glycolic acid solution applied. The low percentage in cosmetic creams and moisturisers has a minimal effect, but stronger solutions (50–70%) can be applied by your dermatologist as a light cosmetic peel. The advantage gained by inducing this type of peel is to encourage minor surface blemishes to slough off—blemishes like the dry blotchy patches in sun damaged skin, superficial seborrhoeic keratoses, solar keratoses, and blotchy superficial pigmentation. Blackheads can be significantly improved, though they will tend to reform.

Glycolic acid works by dissolving the biological glue that holds together the topmost cells of the epidermis, allowing them to slough off more easily. Normally these cells or clumps of them are shed constantly as dry flakes which are invisible to the naked eye. Speeding up the process of sloughing gives the skin a healthy glow and if the peeling process is repeated at intervals, some superficial blemishes like the blotchy pigmentation in sun damaged skin will be improved.

'Exfoliation' is a trendy term often used in cosmetic advertisements. 'Cleanse, tone and nourish' is being superseded by 'cleanse, exfoliate and moisturise', because glycolic acid has gained respectability in the medical profession and cosmetic companies have not been slow to jump on the band wagon. But how many normal skins need to exfoliate? The answer is practically none! As stated previously, our skin exfoliates continually, with dead cells dropping off the surface as new cells move up from the lower layers to replace them.

Red faces

'Broken capillaries' (**telangiectases**) on the cheeks and nose are very common in ageing and sun-damaged skin. They are more likely to occur in fair-skinned people, particularly those with a Celtic background. A note of caution! They may also be a sign of certain skin diseases, so a dermatologist should be consulted before treatment.

Broken capillaries are not actually broken but consist of very small blood vessels just under the surface of the skin which dilate and become visible, mainly because of damage to the supportive tissues and thinning of the epidermis with age. With ageing, some broken capillaries are inevitable on the face, which has a rich network of capillaries in the dermis. Alcohol can make existing capillaries more prominent through a flushing effect, but the so-called 'drinker's nose' is a myth.

If you have this problem and are bothered by it, there are a number of options. Fine wire needle diathermy is one method of eradicating them. In this technique, the small vessel is cauterised with an electric current given through a very fine needle. This causes the blood vessel to shrivel and disappear. No residual scarring occurs if it is done correctly. It is a painful procedure but a topical anaesthetic cream can be applied if necessary. There will be redness in the first few days after treatment and tiny scabs will form. The redness is temporary and will fade in four to seven days. It is easily concealed with foundation. The number of treatments depends on the severity of the condition. An average case might require three to four treatments before a good cosmetic result is achieved. Some laser techniques are also suitable for removing these blemishes (see chapter 10). Another option is simply to camouflage them with appropriate make-up, usually with a green or white tint.

Leg veins

Spider veins on the legs respond best to a technique called sclerotherapy, a treatment in which a 20 per cent salt solution or other fluid is injected under magnification into the veins through a very fine needle. The solution causes irritation of the lining of the vessels, gradually obliterating them over the following four to six weeks. Several treatments may be needed, and support stockings should be worn for at least a week after treatment. There is some discomfort, usually a tingling feeling, and cramps can occur during or just after the injection. Side effects are minor as a rule. The most common is temporary pigmentation which disappears within a month in most cases but may last longer if your skin is naturally heavily pigmented. Very rarely, small superficial ulcers or sores occur at the spot where the injection was given, due to the salt solution pooling in the tissues, and these heal with a small scar.

Peeling procedures to improve the texture of the skin

Light peels employ a high concentration of glycolic acid (50–70%). During the peel a hot tingling sensation is felt and the face becomes slightly pink. There may be some tenderness a few hours after the peel and a little visible flaking is noted over the following days. These peels can be repeated every two to three weeks on four or five occasions, or more often if desired. They are for scaly, blotchy, sun-damaged skin and also keep blackheads at bay in younger skin.

Medium chemical peels are performed using trichloroacetic acid in varying strengths, and they are recommended for skin which is moderately to severely sun damaged, especially if there is a tendency to form multiple keratoses. Within two to three days the superficial layers of the skin begin to turn dark brown and will begin to shed or peel off on the fourth to fifth day. Most people look presentable by the seventh to tenth day after the peel. Sun avoidance is essential after peeling procedures and you should always apply sunscreen. Scarring can result from a medium peel so great care and expertise is needed and aftercare instructions must be followed to the letter.

Deeper peels use chemicals such as phenol which penetrate much more deeply and are therefore appropriate for more severely sun damaged skin and deeper wrinkles and scars. These peels should always be undergone under correct medical supervision because side effects like scarring, excess pigment or loss of pigment can occur. These peels need to be performed in an operating theatre with special equipment to constantly monitor heart rate and blood pressure. They are obviously not undertaken lightly, without the patient first being given a thorough explanation of the risks involved. There is a risk of scarring with all procedures. Some people will scar from minimum injury. The deeper the peel or

procedure, the greater the risk. Some people scar unpre-
dictably and an area of skin should be tested before more
extensive peeling is done.

Dermabrasion

Dermabrasion is a process in which the skin surface is phys-
ically removed by a technique which is rather like sandpa-
pering. It removes the outer layer of the skin (the epidermis)
and the upper portion of the underlying dermis. After this,
new skin cells regenerate to cover the denuded surface. The
new skin tends to look smoother and less blemished.

Dermabrasion is used to improve acne scarring and will
completely eliminate small superficial scars. It is also used to
improve sun damaged skin and will remove superficial spots
and blemishes including solar keratoses (sun spots). It will
also improve wrinkles and completely remove the more
superficial lines. It will not remove dilated capillaries. Dermabrasion can be used to improve surgical scars and scars
from injuries to make them less conspicuous. It has also been
used to remove tattoos, but new lasers are possibly a better
option. Satisfactory tattoo removal remains a problem and
there is no ideal method as yet.

Dermabrasion requires great care and skill on the part of
the operator to avoid scarring and to achieve the desired
improvement without leaving too much of a demarcation
between the treated and untreated areas. To avoid the latter,
it is usually recommended that the full face, or at least a
large area, is dermabraded at one time. In the case of wrinkling around the lips, it is quite common for just this area to
be dermabraded. Some acne patients have scarring on the
cheeks only and occasionally dermabrasion is limited to this
area.

Dermabrasion is usually carried out under general or local
anaesthetic with sedating and pain-relieving drugs given as
required. The skin to be treated is prepared in various ways
just before the dermabrasion is carried out. After the treatment dressings are applied and healing takes approximately
two weeks.

Possible complications include scarring, as mentioned. The other main complication is pigmentation, which is more likely to occur in people with naturally darker skin. In many cases it is temporary and can usually be corrected by using a bleaching cream and avoiding sun exposure. Occasionally, infection is a problem; the main concern is the cold sore virus, or herpes, which can be spread by dermabrasion. All patients with a history of cold sores should have an anti-viral agent called acyclovir to prevent this complication.

Fillers—collagen for recontouring

Injectable collagen comes from the skin of cows. It goes through a treatment and purification process which virtually eliminates all chance of allergy, although anyone contemplating having collagen injections should have an allergy test one month before treatment.

Injectable collagen can be used to improve facial lines and grooves caused by loss of resilience and elasticity as a result of sun damage and natural ageing. It can also be used to give more definition to the lip (this treatment is called the 'Paris Lip'). In this technique the collagen is injected along the lip line to plump it out. It can also be used to highlight the ridges that extend from the upper lip to the nose in the midline, giving the fuller look that is so fashionable these days. It is also useful for filling acne scars or scars following chicken pox, injury or surgery. It can improve frown lines and the deep grooves which run from the nose to the corners of the mouth. Different types of collagen are used depending on the site to be treated. The collagen is injected through a tiny needle into the topmost layers of the skin and there is usually little discomfort. If necessary, local anaesthetic can be used. The main drawback of collagen is its expense and the fact that the benefits are not permanent. Most patients will need periodic re-treatments to maintain the improvement because the collagen is gradually reabsorbed.

There is a great variety of procedures and practitioners available, so shop around and get all the advice you can. Always ask about risks. Ask other consumers as well.

Understand your own expectations and make sure you communicate them to your doctor. Remember that your expectations should be realistic.

THE BOTTOM LINE

It should be stressed that if a woman is satisfied with her appearance and not bothered by minor blemishes or the effect of ageing and photoageing, then so be it! On the other hand, modern cosmetic dermatology provides ways to improve on nature for any woman who wishes to avail herself of it.

CHAPTER TEN

LIGHT YEARS AHEAD

Lasers for skin problems

ANNE HOWARD

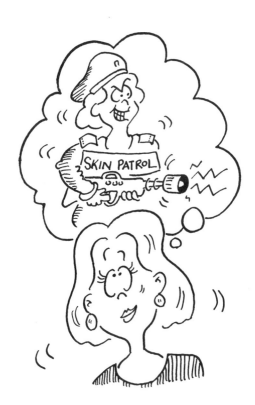

WHAT IS A LASER?

Lasers are powerful and finely focused beams of light. There are lasers which are little more than thin torches—such as the pointer beams used by lecturers—which operators claim can stimulate wound healing, help hair growth and so on. Beware of these! In general there is no proof that they do what they are claimed to do although you will almost certainly waste your money in discovering this. Most medical lasers are extremely expensive pieces of equipment so that few doctors have one in their surgery. Some people expect them to perform miracles such as eradicating skin spots without leaving any mark at all or even removing scars completely. They are certainly very useful machines but they do have limitations!

A laser operator should have a certificate of proof of training. Most work in groups in order to share the cost of the equipment or else are dealing so often in cosmetic work that owning one becomes cost-effective.

The way each laser works depends on the **wavelength,** or colour, of the light which it emits. Light from yellow lasers for instance is taken up by red blood cells, and helps remove red marks. Green light lasers help brown marks, and long wavelength light lasers burn up tissue so they can be used as scalpels which seal the blood vessels as they cut.

There are different lasers for different jobs—there is no *single* magic wand.

LASERS FOR RED MARKS

Yellow-light lasers emit light of a wavelength which is absorbed by haemoglobin, the red pigment in blood. This light can destroy the extra red blood vessels present in some birthmarks. It can also remove unsightly fine vessels which appear with age and too much sun exposure.

Red birthmarks

The most common red birthmark is known as a port wine stain. It is present at birth and grows darker and sometimes thicker with age. It consists of extra blood vessels very close to the surface of the skin. Very light pink birthmarks, sometimes known as stork marks, occur around the eyes and nose and the back of the neck, but disappear over the first few months of life and do not need to be treated. (See chapter 1.)

The larger, pinker or redder permanent birthmarks can now be treated by yellow laser. Marks on the face usually respond best to laser treatment, and of course are the ones which worry the parents most. The best laser for this is a **flash lamp pumped dye tuneable laser**.

With this type of laser a very brief flash of strong yellow light is emitted, targetting the extra blood vessels in the skin and causing them to 'burst'. Because the flash is so rapid, there is not enough time for heat to escape into the surrounding tissues and destroy them, so there is little chance of scarring. The burst blood vessels are gradually taken up by the body's excellent scavenging and cleaning system. Multiple flashes are used for each treatment. A treated area ends up looking like a black or dark purple bruise for a couple of weeks but this eventually fades.

Treatment can begin after about 6 months of age. Psychologically it is often better to treat birthmarks on the face before the child goes to school. Many treatments of the same area are required, and it is rare for the mark to disappear entirely. At best a lightening of 80 to 90 per cent will occur after 6 to 10 treatments. Children usually need a general anaesthetic as the treatment is painful.

Adults with this type of birthmark can also be treated and usually do not need a general anaesthetic. Sometimes an anaesthetic cream is used beforehand. Thick, dark adult port wine stains may not respond as well as those of children to the pulsed yellow dye laser, but other lasers may be suitable. The **argon** laser used to be in fashion but caused too many scars. The **copper vapour laser**, traces out blood vessels and is good for the lumps which sometimes develop in birthmarks. The **KTP laser** and the **krypton laser** will sometimes benefit these darker, thicker marks if they fail to respond to the pulsed yellow dye laser.

'Burst blood vessels'

The extra blood vessels (telangiectases) which appear on people's faces either as a solitary spider-like blemish or as multiple fine wavy lines on the cheeks and nose may be a cosmetic problem. They may respond well to a simple electric current treatment known as fine wire diathermy (see chapter 9). The **argon laser**, the **copper vapour laser**, the **KTP** and **Krypton lasers** and the **pulsed yellow dye laser** can all be used to treat these with good results and minimal scarring—often none. If you want to have this problem treated you should consult a dermatologist or trained laser specialist to find out which is the best method for you. 'Spider veins' on the legs are quite different. They respond poorly to laser therapy and are best treated by injections—sclerotherapy (see chapter 9).

Strawberry marks

A peculiar type of 'birthmark' appears sometimes in children around the age of 2 to 3 months, first as a flat pink or red mark, then later protruding out of the skin like a small strawberry. If left alone it usually eventually disappears all by itself, but it is best to consult a doctor early on about this. Sometimes flash lamp pumped dye tuneable laser treatment very early on will stop it from developing and this may be important when the strawberry mark is growing near the eyes, nose or mouth. (See chapter 1.)

LASERS FOR TATTOOS

Many people have tattoos which they come to regret and badly want to have removed. There has been a long list of treatments which have been tried over the years for tattoo removal, many causing unacceptable scars. The best treatment at present is laser treatment. In general the best type of laser for this purpose is the **Q switched YAG laser**. The **Q switched ruby laser** is an earlier version which is also useful. The laser beam is taken up by the pigment, which disintegrates and is then removed by the body's scavenging system.

Amateur tattoos which are fairly high up in the skin and usually blue-black are the easiest to treat. Once again it must be emphasised that as a rule multiple treatments are needed. Multi-coloured intricate professional tattoos are more difficult to treat. Green and light blue pigments are the most difficult to eradicate with the Q switched YAG or ruby lasers. Unwanted cosmetic tattoo pigment implants, such as eyeliner, eyebrows and liplines, can also be removed or modified with Q switched laser treatment.

It is best to contact your doctor or dermatologist for advice on where to have treatment. As mentioned these sophisticated lasers are extremely expensive, so few doctors have them. As there is no Medicare rebate for tattoo removal, treatment is costly, but most people end up satisfied. The procedure is uncomfortable but not very painful—probably less painful than acquiring the tattoo in the first place. The psychological benefit usually far outweighs the discomfort entailed.

LASERS FOR CUTTING AND DESTROYING

The **carbon dioxide laser** emits light of a long wavelength, longer than visible light, in the infrared range. If a broad flat beam is used the laser can be used to destroy various skin lumps, including warts. If a fine narrow beam is used the laser will cut through tissue like a knife, but with no bleeding. More recently the **Superpulse CO_2 laser** and now the **Ultrapulse CO_2 laser** have become available. These are claimed to give the operators better and finer control.

Often there is very little advantage in using such complicated and expensive tools rather than a simple scalpel. On the face, however, in the removal of small lumps or operating near the eye it is better if there is not too much bleeding, because it not only looks unsightly but can delay healing.

Currently, carbon dioxide lasers are used for treating sun damaged lips, removing some surface growths, removing bags around the eyes (blepharoplasty), and fining down wrinkles. Do not expect your doctor or dermatologist to necessarily have one of these machines available. Other methods of treatment may be just as effective and are usually much less expensive.

LASERS FOR BROWN MARKS

Brown marks on the skin are often caused by too much sun exposure. If there is a slightest suspicion that a brown mark is a skin cancer or melanoma, it should **never** be treated by laser. Green light lasers which include certain settings of the KTP, Krypton and Q switched YAG laser can help remove some benign brown marks such as freckles. They also may help melasma—the brown blotches on the face common in women taking the pill and during pregnancy. As a rule it is best to try other treatments including depigmenting creams or liquid nitrogen cryotherapy first, as many cases respond well to these simpler and less costly measures.

SUMMARY

In summary the laser is a useful medical tool—not a magic wand! Correct training in its use is vital if success is to be achieved. You should be wary of laser operators who promise unrealistic results since the treatments they offer will usually be ineffective as well as expensive. Newer and better lasers will continue to be developed as technology advances.

INDEX

Aborigines 23
acne 37–54
  aggravating factors 21, 43, 47, 87, 141, 161, 165
  and hirsutism 61, 85, 91
  blackheads 20, 40, 41, 42–3, 45, 46, 48, 73, 161, 165, 167, 171
  in adolescence 21–3, 38–53
  duration in women 43–4
  make-up and moisturisers 47–8
  myths 21, 42–3
  role of hormones 20, 38–41, 44
  treatment 22, 44–53
    antibiotics 48–50
    cleaning skin 21, 44–5, 73
    oral contraceptives 50–2, 54, 62, 64–5, 73, 74
    Ro-Accutane (oral isotretinoin) 50–1, 53, 74
    topical applications 45–7
      antibiotic lotions 46
      azaleic acid 46

  benzoyl peroxide 22, 45–6
  isotretinoin 46, 50–1, 53, 74
  sulfur, salicylic acid and resorcinol 45, 47
  tretinoin 46, 169–70
  value of medication 22–3
  in babies 20–1
  in children 19–23, 43
    causes 20–1
    myths 21
    treatment 21–2
  in menopausal women 62, 64, 71, 73–6
  in older women 44, 53–4
  in pregnancy 42, 51, 67
  oily skin 38, 40, 45, 54
  pre-menstrual 40, 53–4, 65
  scarring 21, 44, 48
    scar types 52–3
    treatment
      cortisone and collagen injections 53, 175–6
      dermabrasion 53, 174–5
      skin peels 53

types
  acne vulgaris   40–1
  cystic acne   40, 41, 44, 50–1,
    52, 74
  whiteheads   167–8
adolescence   37–56
  changes in birthmarks   5
  Cushing's Syndrome   69
  female genital mutilation   105
  hair growth at puberty   39–40,
    59, 84
  hormonal changes   39–40
    passim, 54
  onset of menstruation   40
  sweating   54–6
  see also acne
advertising   60, 87, 159, 160–3
  passim
Africans   23, 96
ageing   vi
  acne in older women   44, 53–4
  ageing skin   168–9
  benign blemishes   77, 167–8,
    171
  bruising   76
  candida and thrush   76–7
  collagen degeneration   76
  hair loss   77, 91
  incontinence   112–13
  intertrigo   76–7
  lichen sclerosus (LS)   113–14
  ridged nails   77, 129
  seborrhoeic keratosis   66, 70,
    76, 167
  skin cancer   76, 148
  skin in elderly women   76–8
  skin tags with weight gain   76
  solar lentigines (liver spots)   76,
    144, 167
  sweating   76, 77
  vulval pain   119
  wrinkles   72, 162–3, 168–9,
    174–5
  see also menopause; photoageing

AIDS   107
Aldactone   54
allergies
  allergens   32, 110
  in children   18, 31–3
  patch testing   111, 139
  to benzoyl peroxide   45–6
  to cosmetics   32, 73, 139, 164,
    166
  to industrial chemicals   32
  to nail products   130–1, 139
  to sunscreens   25, 26
  to tetracyclines   49
  see also eczema; insects; plant
    allergies; urticaria
alopecia *see* hair loss
alternative therapies *see* natural
  therapies
anorexia   58, 62
anti-androgens
  cyproterone acetate   54, 62–3,
    65, 74, 85, 91
  spironolactone   62–3, 74, 85,
    91
antibiotics
  and dermatitis   10, 110, 135
  as cause of thrush   107
  effect on oral contraceptives
    64–5
  for acne   48–50, 49
  for impetigo   34
  for nail conditions   128
  for rosacea   75
  tetracyclines   48–50, 64
antihistamines
  as cause of allergic contact
    dermatitis   110
  for eczema   10
  for hives   33
  for insect bites   31
  for itchy skin   68
arthritis   13
Asians   6, 23, 59, 96, 103, 150
asthma   6, 134

athlete's foot *see* tinea
Australasian College of
  Dermatologists 155

babies
  susceptibility to sun 23–4
  use of sunscreens 26
  see also acne; birthmarks; cradle
    cap; eczema; nappy rash
baldness *see* hair loss
Billings method 106
birthmarks 2–6
  camouflage make-up 166
  risks of malignancy 5–6
  treatment 2
    laser 4–5, 178–80 *passim*
    surgical 5–6
  types
    blood vessel 2–5
      port wine stains (capillary
        malformation) 4–5, 166,
        179
      stork marks (naevus
        flammeus) 3, 179
      strawberry marks
        (haemangioma) 3–4, 180
    pigmentation 5–6
      brown birthmarks (congenital
        melanocytic naevi) 5–6
      Mongolian spots 6
blackheads *see* acne
body odour 54–5, 106
  {see also} sweating
broken capillaries 65, 67–8, 75,
  77, 168, 171–4 *passim*
  camouflage make-up 166–7
  treatment 68, 171–4 *passim*,
    180
  see also birthmarks; photoageing
bulimia 62

Campbell de Morgan spots 77
cancer 5–6, 88, 116
  see also skin cancer

carcinoma
  basal cell carcinoma (BCC) 146
    development 146
    treatment 146
      diagnotic biopsy 147
      liquid nitrogen 147
      Moh's micrographic surgery
        147
      skin curette 147
      surgery 146–7 *passim*
    types
      morphoeic (fibrosing) 146
      nodulo-ulcerative 146
      pigmented 146
      superficial 147
  squamous cell carcinoma (SCC)
    148
    risk categories 148
    treatment
      radiotherapy 148
      surgical removal 148
cataracts 143
child sexual abuse
  genital conditions as indicators
    11, 116
children 1–36
  children's skin vi, 39–40
  effect of sun 143, 168
  nail biting 128
  see also acne; babies; child sexual
    abuse; eczema; herpes;
    impetigo; insects; moles; plant
    allergies; psoriasis; sun
    protection; tinea; urticaria;
    warts
chloasma *see* pigmentation
clothing
  and dermatitis 8, 110, 111,
    137
  and nail problems 126, 128,
    129
  disposable v. cloth nappies
    18–19
  protective clothing

against insects   31
against sun   24–5
support stockings   172
underwear   77, 112, 122
cold sores *see* herpes
collagen   ix, 53, 76, 175–6
contact dermatitis   133–40
allergic   135–40
non-occupational triggers
130, 136, 139
occupational triggers   137–9
risk occupations   137
symptoms   135
testing   8–9, 136, 139
treatment   140
eyelid dermatitis   166
from hormone replacement
therapy patches   76
irritant   133–5
acute v. chronic   133
prevention and treatment
7–10, 134–5
risk occupations   134–5
triggers   7–8, 133–4
vulval   109–11
symptoms   109
table of allergens   110
table of irritants   110
treatment
avoidance of irritants and
allergens   110–11
cortisone creams   111
patch testing   111
salt bathing   111
see also plant allergies
contact urticaria *see* urticaria
contraceptives   106, 110
see also oral contraceptives
cortisone
corticosteroids   59, 85
for forms of dermatitis   9–10,
75, 111, 135
for hair loss   90
for insect bites in children   31

for lichen sclerosus   114
for nappy rash   19
for psoriasis   84
for strawberry birthmarks   4
for treatment of plant allergies in
children   32
injections for acne scarring   53
cosmetics   160–8 *passim*
and acne   21, 43, 47, 73, 165
as allergens   73, 121, 136, 139,
165–6
beauty culture   vi, 59–60, 60,
159
camouflage make-up   159,
166–7
cleansing products   160–1
improving on nature   165–8
make-up   166
masks and facials   164–5
moisturisers   47, 161–5 *passim*,
171
and wrinkles   162–3
needed only for dryness   163
pseudoscientific claims   162–3
psychological benefits   164
see also nails; sunscreens
cradle cap   10–11
causes   10, 13
treatment   11
cryotherapy   70, 116, 144–5,
147, 167
Cushing's Syndrome   69
Cyclosporin A   85

dandruff   11, 83, 84
Depo-Provera   108
dermabrasion   53, 174–5
dermatitis *see* eczema
diabetes   107
diathermy   70, 116, 167, 172
diet   14, 21, 22, 42, 55, 89, 92,
107, 109
drugs
anaesthetics   92, 110, 172

anticancer   88, 144, 152
anti-epilepsy   43
antifungal   35, 108, 127–9
   passim
anti-inflammatory   128
Depo-Provera   108
fluconazole   108
immuno-suppressant   107
ketoconazole   108
lithium   43
metronidazole   75
minoxidil   59
   Regaine   91
nystatin   108
steroids   43, 59, 85, 135
tretinoin and isotretinoin   46,
   63–4, 69, 74, 169–70
   Ro-Accutane   50–1, 53, 74
tricyclic antidepressants   119
zinc pirithione   83, 84
see also anti-androgens;
   antibiotics; antihistamines;
   cortisone; hormone
   replacement therapy; oral
   contraceptives; topical
   applications; vitamins and
   minerals

eczema   viii
   effect of pregnancy   69
   in children   6–10
      allergy testing   8–9
      irritants   7–8
      skin care   9–10
      symptoms   6–7
      treatment   7–10
         cortisone creams   9–10
   in menopausal women   72
   peri-oral dermatitis   75
   resemblance to skin cancer   147
   see also contact dermatitis;
      cradle cap; nappy rash;
      psoriasis; seborrhoeic
      dermatitis

ethnic women   6, 23, 59, 60, 81,
   96, 103, 105, 150
exfoliation   161, 171

facial hair *see* hirsutism
5-fluorouracil   144
fleas   30
fluconazole   108
fungal infections
   and occupational disease   141
   see also nails; tinea

genital skin problems   100–23
   common skin diseases of vulva
      101
   enlargement of clitoris and hair
      loss   91
   female genital mutilation   105
   incontinence   112–13, 122
   normal secretions   104, 121
   normal vaginal discharge
      105–6
      Billings method of cervical
         mucus examinations   106
      effects of the Pill   105
      menstrual cycle   105–6
   ovarian tumours   61
   sore sex   119
   structure of external genital area
      101–5 *passim*
   terminology   102, 122
   vulval biopsy   112, 119–20
   vulval hygiene   120–2
      and incontinence   122
      cotton underwear   122
      Pap smear   122, 123
      self-examination   122
   vulval itching   106–7
   vulval malignant melanoma
      150
   vulval pain   118–19
      essential vulvodynia   119
      tampon or intercourse
         sensitivity   119

treatment
 tricyclic antidepressants 119
 vulvar vestibulitis 119
what is normal 101–5
 description of normal vagina
  104–5
 guide to self-examination 102
 menstrual pain 103–4
 see also eczema; intertrigo; lichen
 sclerosus (LS); moles; nappy
 rash; psoriasis; sexually
 transmissible diseases (STD);
 thrush; warts
gingivitis 68
golden staph 34
Greer, Germaine 75, 78

haemorrhoids 68
hair viii, 79–99
 changes at puberty 39–40, 59,
  84
 dandruff 11, 83, 84
 dreadlocks 98
 effects of pregnancy 70
 growth cycle 81–3
 hair products
  colouring products 94–6
  hair extensions 97
  permanent waving solutions
   96–7
  shampoos and conditioners
   93–4
  straighteners 97
 improvement during pregnancy
  67
 itchy scalp 83
 long hair and acne 42
 psoriasis
  symptoms 83, 84
  treatment 83, 84
 seborrhoeic dermatitis
  causes 83–4
  treatment 83, 84
 structure 80–2
 trichologists and hair clinics
  98–9

types 81, 96
 see also hair loss; hirsutism;
  hypertrichosis; nails; skin
hair loss (alopecia) 87–93
 alopecia areata (AA) 89–90
  and nail changes 90
  and stress 89
  autoimmune phenomenon 89
  in children 89
  treatment 90
 androgenetic alopecia (MPA) 39,
  71, 80, 89, 90–1
  and oral contraceptives 65,
   92–3
  causes 90–1
  treatment
   anti-androgens 91
   Regaine 91
 in old age 77
 non-scarring alopecia 88–9
  causes 88
  reversible 88
 scarring alopecia 87–8
  scalp biopsies 88
 telogen effluvium (increased
  shedding) 92
hay fever 6, 134
head lice (nits)
 in children 27–8
  concurrent with impetigo 34
  contagious 28
  life cycle 27–8
  treatment 28
herpes
 cold sores 117
 genital herpes 117–18
 in children 35–6, 117
  causes 35
  sites 35
  symptoms 36
  treatment 36
 types 117
hirsutism 58–63, 91
 and virilisation 61, 85
 at menopause 53, 62, 71, 73,
  74

causes
    androgen hormones   38–9,
        58–61, 73, 74, 84–5
    hereditary   60
    defined   58, 84
    ethnic variations   59, 60
    notions of normality   59–60,
        62, 84–5
    psychological aspects   61–2, 74
    relation to acne   61, 85, 91
    sites   84
    treatment   61–3, 62
        anti-androgens   62–3, 74, 85
        camouflage   62, 74, 86
        depilation   85–6
        epilation   86–7
            electrolysis and thermolysis
                63, 86
            shaving   86
            waxing   61, 63
    see also hypertrichosis
hives see urticaria
hormone replacement therapy
    (HRT) see menopause
hormones   x, 57–78
    and pilo-sebaceous unit   20,
        38–41, 44, 73
    endocrine gland   38–40 passim
    role of hormones and skin
        38–40
    sex hormones
        androgens   20, 38–41 passim,
            54, 58, 59, 60–3 passim,
            70–1, 73, 84–5, 90–1
        oestrogen and progesterone
            38, 91
    sweat glands   54
    see also acne; anti-androgens;
        hair; hirsutism; hormone
        replacement therapy;
        menopause; menstruation; oral
        contraceptives; pregnancy
hot flushes   66, 71
hypertrichosis   58–9, 84
    causes
        anorexia   58

corticosteroid drugs   59, 85
    minoxidil   59
    see also hirsutism
hysterectomy   62

immune system   12, 32, 69, 88,
    89, 107, 116, 148
impetigo (school sores)
    in children   33–4
        causes   33
            golden staph   33–4
            infectious   33
            symptoms   33–4
            treatment with antibiotics   34
incontinence   112–13, 122
Indians   23
insects
    and children   30–1
        fleas   30
        mosquitoes   30
        paspalum mite   30–1
        prevention   31
            repellents and protective
                clothing   31
        treatment
            antihistamines   31
            calamine lotion and cortisone
                creams   31
    see also head lice; scabies
intertrigo
    and childbirth   112
    and incontinence   112–13
    and menopause   112
    and sweating   76
    associated with thrush   76–7
    treatment   77
iron deficiencies   89, 107
itchy scalp   83

ketoconazole   108
kidney disease   88, 148

laser therapy   167, 177–82
    and skin cancer   182
    brown marks   182
    definitions   178

functions   181–2
laser types   178–82 *passim*
red marks   178–80 *passim*
  birthmarks   4–5, 178–80
  broken capillaries   172
  burst blood vessels   180
  low scarring   179
tattoos   174, 180–1
treatment of children   179
lice *see* head lice
lichen sclerosus (LS)   101,
  113–14
  and skin cancer   114
  changes in labia minora   113
  in children   114
  itching   113
  not confined to older women
    114–15
  treatment   114
liquid nitrogen *see* cryotherapy
liver spots   76, 144, 167
lupus erythematosus   69, 88

malignant melanoma *see*
  melanoma
medication *see* drugs, topical
  applications
Mediterraneans   59, 60, 103
melanoma   viii
  and children   15, 16
  and vulval moles   115
  high incidence in Australia   16,
    23
  malignant melanoma   148–52
  and moles   14–17 *passim*, 16,
    23, 115, 149–50 *passim*
  and sun exposure   148
  early removal and high survival
    rates   148–9
  five stages   151
  treatment   152
    surgical removal   152
    vaccines   152
  types
    acral lentiginous   150

in lining of eye, mouth and
  vulva   150
lentigo maligna (Hutchinson's
  melanotic freckle)   150
nodular   150
superficial spreading
  149–50
warning signs   151
melasma *see* pigmentation
menopause   vi, 70–6 *passim*
  acne   71, 73–6 *passim*
    treatment   64, 73–4
  effect on skin   70–3
  hirsutism   53, 62, 71, 73, 74
  hormonal changes   70–1, 73
  hormone replacement therapy
    (HRT)   71–4 *passim*, 76
    alternative therapies   71
    contact dermatitis from patches
      76
    depigmenting lotions and
      creams   76
    effect on skin   72, 76
    melasma   63, 76
    sun protection   76
  hot flushes   66, 71
  intertrigo   112
  peri-oral dermatitis   75
  rosacea   74–5
  see also hair loss
menstruation
  and vaginal discharge   106
  effect on skin   65–6
  irregularities and hair loss   91
  menstrual cycle   105–6
  menstrual pain   103–4
  onset   40
  pre-menstrual acne   65
  pre-menstrual hot flushes   66
  sanitary napkins as cause of
    vulval dermatitis   110
  tampons and vulval pain   119
metronidazole   75
minerals *see* vitamins and minerals
mites *see* head lice; insects; scabies

moles
  and benign skin lesions 152–4
  and risk of melanoma 15, 16,
    115, 148–50 *passim*, 149, 150
  and sun exposure 23
  appearance 15–17 *passim*
  bleeding 15
  brown birthmarks 5–6
  changes 14–17 *passim*, 66, 148
  genital moles and other brown
    marks 114–15
    after childbirth 114
    and melanoma 115
    dysplastic (atypical) 115
    regular self-examination 115
  halo naevus phenomenon 16
  in children 14–17
  in pregnancy 15
  inspection 16, 115, 150
  normal features 14–17 *passim*
  sun protection 16
  surgical removal 17
  see also skin cancer
Mongolian spots 6
mosquitoes 30

nails viii, 124–31
  affected by psoriasis 13, 129
  brittleness and flaking 126,
    130
  fungal infection 129–30
  ingrown toenails 129
  lifting nails (onycholysis) 90,
    127, 129, 131
  nail biting 128–9
    common in children 128
  nail changes and hair loss 90
  nail cosmetics 130–1
    nail polish removers 126, 130
    polishes 130
      allergic reactions 110, 130,
        139
    synthetic nails 131
  occupational diseases
    (paronychia) 127, 141

ridged nails 77, 129
  structure 125–6
  swollen nail folds (paronychia)
    127–8
  warts around nails 11
  white lines 128
  see also hair; skin
nappy rash 13, 17–19
  aggravating factors 18
  and development of thrush
    17–18
  and psoriasis 18
  treatment 18–19
    allergies to treatment 18
    and teething 18
    and thrush 17–18
    cloth v. disposable nappies
      18–19
    cortisone and anti-infective
      creams 19
    keep clean, dry and cool
      18–19
natural therapies 10, 12, 71, 163
Negroids 81, 96
nickel 110, 137
nits *see* head lice

occupational health 132–41
  passim
oral contraceptives 92–3
  and hair loss 65, 92–3
  Diane 35 ED 52, 65, 74
  effect of antibiotics 49–50, 64,
    64–5
  effect on skin 63–5
  effect on vaginal discharge
    105–6
  for hirsutism 62–3
  for menopausal women 74, 75
  levonorgestrol 64–5
  pigmentation of the face
    (melasma) 63–4, 66
  treatment
    glycolic acid 64

hydroquinone and
isotretinoin 63–4
sun protection 64
spiders 65
telogen effluvium on ceasing 92
thrush 64
treatment of acne 50–2, 54, 62,
64–5, 73, 74

Pap smears 116, 122, 123
paspalum mite 30–1
peeling procedures 144, 161,
169–71, 173–4
pets 8, 30, 34
photoageing 72, 143–5, 167–76
passim
and sun lamps 42
and sunscreens 155
definition 143
effect on skin structure 143
in children 143
effects 76
Bowen's disease 144
broken capillaries
(telangiectases) 143, 168,
174
brown spots 143
liver spots (solar lentigines)
144
premature ageing 143
solar keratoses 144, 174
wrinkling 143, 168, 174
minimal effect of cosmetics
162–3
treatment 169–76
cryosurgery with liquid
nitrogen 144–5
dermabrasion 53, 174–5
exfoliation 161, 171
injectable collagen 175–6
peeling procedures 144, 161,
169–70, 171, 173–4
surgical removal 144
tretinoin 169–70
see also skin cancer

pigmentation ix, 53, 168
and skin types 23, 66
as sun protection 23
depigmenting lotions and creams
76
effect of sunlight 63
of the face (melasma, chloasma)
and menopause 76
and oral contraceptives 63–4,
66
during pregnancy 63–4, 66–7
treatment 63–4, 171
see also birth marks
Pill, the *see* oral contraceptives
pimples *see* acne
plant allergies 31–2, 137
compositae dermatitis 138
grevillea ('Robyn Gordon')
31–2, 138
in children 31–2
rhus 31, 138
symptoms 31
treatment 32
plastic surgery 159
liposuction 159
remodelling 159
pollens 33
pregnancy 66–70
acne 42, 44, 51, 67
cracked nipples 69
disruption of hymen 104
effect of drugs
Ro-Accutane 50
tetracyclines 49
tretinoin 46
effect on auto-immune diseases
69
effect on psoriasis and eczema
69
effects on hair 67, 70, 92
episiotomies 104
haemorrhoids 68
herpes 118
itchy skin 68
other skin problems 67–70

skin pigmentation   66–7
  and pigment-stimulating
    hormones   66–7
  changes in moles   15, 66
  melasma   63–4, 66
  seborrhoeic keratoses   66, 70,
    76, 167
skin tags   70
spiders   65, 67, 68
stretch marks   68, 69
  and Cushing's Syndrome   69
  isotretinoin creams   69
  myths   69
swollen red gums   68
thrush   107
varicose veins   68
vulval moles after childbirth
  114
psoriasis
  and hot flushes   66
  as cause of cradle cap   10, 11
  as occupational disease   141
  different in adults and children
    13
  effect of pregnancy   69
  genital   13, 111–12
    biopsy   112
  hereditary   13
  in adults   13
  in children   2, 13–14
    and nappy rash   18
  on scalp   84
    cortisone creams and lotions
      84
    specialised creams and
      shampoos   84
    symptoms   83, 84
    tar   84
    vitamin D cream   84
  resemblance to skin cancer   147
  see also eczema
puberty see adolescence

radiotherapy   148
Regaine   91

ringworm see tinea
Ro-Accutane (oral isotretinoin)
  50–1, 53, 74
rosacea   74–5
rubber   137, 141

scabies
  in children   28–30
    allergic reactions   28
    concurrent with impetigo   34
    contagious   28–9
    life cycle   28
    treatment   29–30
      lindane and permethrin
        creams   29–30
scalp
  and pilo-sebaceous unit   38, 39
  biopsies   88
  see also cradle cap; hair;
    psoriasis; tinea
scaly scalp see cradle cap
scarring
  acne   21, 44, 48, 52–3, 174
    scar types   52–3
  after surgery for sweating   56
  epilation   87
  episiotomies   104
  low scarring in laser therapy
    179
  removal of moles   17
  removal of warts   12
  surgical scars and broken
    capillaries   174
  vulval moles around surgical
    scars   114
school sores see impetigo
sclerotherapy   172–3
seborrhoeic dermatitis   83
  and dandruff   83
  as cause of cradle cap   10
  in genital skin   110
seborrhoeic ketatoses   66, 70, 76,
  167
self-examination
  and vulval hygiene   122

Billings method of cervical
  mucus examination 106
for sun damage 150
genital 102
of moles 16, 115
of vaginal discharge 122
Semitic women 59, 60
sexual abuse *see* child sexual abuse
sexual intercourse 105, 106,
  108, 111, 112, 119–21 *passim*
  see also sexually transmissible
  diseases
sexually transmissible diseases
  115–18
  chlamydia 115
  genital conditions in children
    11, 114, 116
  gonorrhoea 115
  pubic lice (crabs) 115
  specialised clinics 118
  syphilis 115
  see also genital skin problems;
    herpes; warts
skin vi–xi
  changes in puberty 38–40, 51
  changes through ageing 168
  effect of sun 143, 168
  external genital area 101–2
  of children vi, 39–40, 143, 168
  pilo-sebaceous unit x, 20,
    38–41, 73
  structure vii–x, 133
  see also hair; hormones; nails;
    pigmentation
skin cancer vi, 42, 145–52
  passim
  and lichen sclerosus 114
  and sun exposure 23
  and sunscreens 26
  as occupational disease 141
  in Australia 23, 27, 143, 145
  malignant lesions 143
  pre-malignant lesions 143

resemblance to Bowen's disease
  147
see also carcinoma; melanoma;
  photoageing; sun damage
skin treatment 158–76
  bleaching creams 167
  cryotherapy 70, 116, 144–5,
    147, 167
  dermabrasion 53, 174–5
  diathermy 70, 116, 167, 172
  exfoliation 161, 171
  injectable collagen 175–6
  peeling procedures 144, 161,
    169–71, 173–4
  sclerotherapy 172–3
  see also cosmetics; laser therapy;
    plastic surgery
smoking 169
solariums 156–7
spiders *see* broken capillaries
stress viii, 14, 21, 43, 54, 55, 74,
  89
stretch marks (striae) 68, 69
sun damage vi, 142–57
  and blackheads and oil cysts
    167
  and skin types 23
  and sun exposure 16
  and sunlight 23
  benign skin lesions 152–4
    moles (naevi)
      compound 153
      dysplastic 153–4
      intradermal 153
      junctional 152–3
  cataract formation 143
  'healthy tan' 24
  photosensitising drugs 46, 50
  self-examination 150
  sensitivity of babies 23–4
  solarium hazards 156–7
  sunburn 35, 42, 143, 145
  sunlamps 42

ultraviolet light   26
see also photoageing;
   pigmentation; skin cancer; sun
   protection
sun protection
   danger times   24, 154–5
   effect of sun on children   143
   for children   2, 16, 23–7, 159
   keeping out of the sun   21, 26,
   154–7
   role of pigmentation   23
   vitamin D   24
   see also sunscreens
sunscreens   24–7, 155–6, 165
   allergic reactions   26, 27, 139
   and cancer   26
   chemical free   26
   fluorescent zinc sticks   27
   for acne   48
   not a cause of cancer   26
   protection policy needed   27
   sun protection factor (SPF)
   25–7
   types   27
surgery
   curettage   67–8, 144, 147
   for basal cell carcinoma   146–7
   Moh's micrographic surgery
      147
   for birthmarks   5–6
   for ingrown toenails   129
   for malignant melanoma   148,
   152
   for moles   17
   for skin cancers   144
   for skin tags   70
   for sweating   55–6
   for warts   12, 70
   see also cryotherapy; laser
      therapy; plastic surgery;
      scarring; skin treatment
sweating   viii
   and hot flushes   71

and intertrigo   76, 112
and sunscreens   25
antiperspirants   55
body odour   54–5
cause of vulval dermatitis   110
hyperhidrosis (excessive
   sweating) 54
in adolescence   54–6
night sweats and menopause   71
sweat glands   x, 54–5, 77
treatment   55–6

tattoos   166, 174, 180–1
teenagers *see* adolescence
telangiectases *see* broken
   capillaries
tetracyclines   48–50, 64
thrush   107–9
   and tetracyclines   49
   as cause of lifting nails   127
   associated with intertrigo   76–7
   causes   64, 107
   in children   17–18
   role of lactobacilli   107
   symptoms   106–7
      uncomfortable sexual
         intercourse   108
      treatment   107–9 *passim*
thyroid   88
tinea
   fungal infection   34, 129
   in adults (athlete's foot)   35
   in children (ringworm)   34–5
titanium   26
tonsillitis   13
topical applications
   antifungal   35, 108
   azaleic acid   46
   benzoyl peroxide   22, 45–6
   glycolic acid   64, 169, 170–1
   hydroquinone   63–4
   insecticide creams   29

lindane and permethrin creams
29–30
local anaesthetics 110
selenium sulfide 83, 84

urticaria
in children 32–3
causes 33
allergens 32–3
viral illness 33
symptoms 32
treatment with antihistamines
33
in the workplace 140–1
allergic reaction 141
prick testing 141
triggers
food 141
rubber 141

vagina *see* genital skin problems
varicose veins 68
vitamins and minerals
and psoriasis 13
iron deficiencies 89, 107
Ro-Accutane for acne 50–1,
53, 74
vitamin D
and sunlight 24
cream for eczema and psoriasis
84
zinc 26, 27, 83, 89
vulva *see* genital skin problems

warts
genital warts 115–16, 118

in children 11–12
Pap smears 116
treatment
as cause of vulval dermatitis
110
chemical paints and plaster
12
diathermy 70, 116
hypnotherapy 12
laser therapy 181
liquid nitrogen therapy 70,
116
natural therapies 12
surgical removal 12, 70
types
filiform 11
plane 11
plantar 11
seborrhoeic keratoses 66, 70,
76, 167
skin tags 76
wart virus infection (HPV)
115–16
as occupational disease 141
causes
depressed immune system
116
human papilloma virus (HPV)
115
workplace 132–41
see also contact dermatitis;
urticaria

zinc 26, 27, 83, 89
zits *see* acne